DOING DIALECTICAL BEHAVIOR THERAPY

Guides to Individualized Evidence-Based Treatment

Jacqueline B. Persons, *Series Editor*

Providing road maps for managing real-world cases, volumes in this series help the clinician develop treatment plans using interventions of proven effectiveness. With an emphasis on systematic yet flexible case formulation, these hands-on guides provide powerful alternatives to one-size-fits-all approaches. Each book addresses a particular disorder or presents cutting-edge intervention strategies that can be used across a range of clinical problems.

Doing Dialectical Behavior Therapy
A PRACTICAL GUIDE

Kelly Koerner

Series Editor's Note by Jacqueline B. Persons

Foreword by Marsha M. Linehan

THE GUILFORD PRESS
New York   London

©2012 The Guilford Press
A Division of Guilford Publications, Inc.
72 Spring Street, New York, NY 10012
www.guilford.com

Printed in the United States of America

This book is printed on acid-free paper.

Last digit is print number: 9   8   7   6   5   4   3   2   1

The author has checked with sources believed to be reliable in her efforts to
provide information that is complete and generally in accord with the standards
of practice that are accepted at the time of publication. However, in view of the
possibility of human error or changes in behavioral, mental health, or medical
sciences, neither the author, nor the editor and publisher, nor any other party
who has been involved in the preparation or publication of this work warrants
that the information contained herein is in every respect accurate or complete,
and they are not responsible for any errors or omissions or the results obtained
from the use of such information. Readers are encouraged to confirm the
information contained in this book with other sources.

**Library of Congress Cataloging-in-Publication Data is available
from the Publisher**

ISBN 978-1-4625-0232-5

In loving dedication to Claire, Tom, SB, and NB

About the Author

Kelly Koerner, PhD, is Founder and Creative Director of the Evidence-Based Practice Institute, where she explores how technology can be used for learning and collaboration to help practitioners get better clinical outcomes. She is an expert clinician, clinical supervisor, and trainer in dialectical behavior therapy (DBT), with specialized training in many other evidence-based treatments. She has served as Director of Training for Marsha M. Linehan's research investigating the efficacy of DBT for suicidal and drug-abusing individuals with borderline personality disorder; Creative Director at Behavioral Tech Research, where she developed e-learning and other technology-based methods to disseminate evidence-based practices; and Co-Founder and first CEO of Behavioral Tech, a company that provides training in DBT. Dr. Koerner is a Clinical Faculty member at the University of Washington and maintains a small clinical consulting practice in Seattle.

Series Editor's Note

Readers are in for a treat. In this book, Kelly Koerner describes in detail the skills needed by the individual therapist who is providing dialectical behavior therapy (DBT) to the complex multiple-problem patient. DBT was originally developed by Marsha M. Linehan at the University of Washington for the treatment of chronic suicidal behavior, and she later extended it to provide treatment to patients who meet criteria for borderline personality disorder and suffer from life-threatening and quality-of-life-threatening behaviors, including suicidality, self-harm, impulsive self-destructive behaviors, tumultuous interpersonal relationships, unemployment, homelessness, and poverty. DBT, when provided in a comprehensive package that includes individual therapy, group skills training, and consultation with the therapist, has been shown in several randomized controlled trials to provide effective treatment for patients who have borderline personality disorder, and recent controlled studies have shown that DBT is also effective for treating substance abuse, bulimia, and binge eating.

When patients have suicidal and self-harm behaviors, intense emotions, impulsive behaviors, uncertainty about their goals and even their identity, and desperate life circumstances—and when all these occur in the context of intense and rapidly shifting emotional states and behaviors—therapists need skilled guidance. DBT and this book can provide it.

Koerner describes the conceptual framework underpinning DBT and provides rich clinical detail that shows the therapist how to use the framework to prioritize and intervene effectively when patients have multiple high-priority targets, as, for example, when the patient in your office at this moment is having strong urges to die, is about to be evicted, and begins dissociating in the session when you step in to try to provide help. These types of situations are challenging in their own right, and arouse high emotions that make it difficult for the therapist to be effective. Clear thinking and sophisticated skills are needed to navigate safely when there are pounding waves and craggy rocks, and Koerner's book provides both.

DBT is complicated, partly because it is so flexible and adaptable to the needs of each patient at each moment. Koerner spells out in detail what is needed to obtain a formulation of the case in DBT, and how to use the formulation to guide intervention.

This book is jam-packed with useful knowledge. I have read it twice and learned from it each time. Koerner provides both a careful account of DBT's conceptual framework and a huge amount of rich clinical detail, and she links the two very skillfully, showing how the general framework and the conceptualization of the case that is founded on the framework guide the therapist's behavior at every moment, especially the most difficult ones.

The richness of this book results, no doubt, in part from the fact that the author is multitalented. Koerner is a consummate expert in DBT, originally trained by Marsha Linehan, and has a deep understanding of the therapy. She is also a skilled consultant to clinicians using DBT and has an empathic understanding of the dilemmas that therapists confront as they use DBT. My experience of Koerner's clinical and interpersonal skills is first-hand: she has been my DBT consultant for several years, and I rely on her for consultation whenever I care for complex and challenging patients. She is also able to write about the therapy, and not all skilled clinicians can do this. She can spell out the understructure of DBT in a way that gives the reader a thoughtful guide to making clinical decisions that are firmly grounded in DBT principles. She is also a highly regarded teacher and trainer with an international reputation. Her clinical, consultation, writing, and teaching skills are on full display here. The result is a book that makes a truly outstanding contribution to the Guides to Individualized Evidence-Based Treatment series.

JACQUELINE B. PERSONS, PhD

Foreword

Kelly Koerner, one of my former students, is a longtime collaborator. She cofounded with me a company whose mission is to make evidence-based treatments available to all individuals with severe mental disorders. Beyond a doubt, she is one of the strongest clinical trainers, supervisors, and writers in the dialectical behavior therapy (DBT) field. I first met Kelly as a second-year graduate student when she joined my clinical practicum in 1989. Those were the days when I would bring the practicum students mimeographed copies of what would become my treatment manual, *Cognitive-Behavioral Treatment of Borderline Personality Disorder*. Kelly and her peers on the graduate student consultation team can best be considered co-creators of the treatment that later became DBT. She and her colleagues soon were among the best trained and most experienced therapists in our area of expertise. Even today, it is extremely difficult to find a clinical supervisor who knows more than Kelly and her colleagues do about treating suicidal behavior.

For the past two decades, Kelly and I have worked closely together in various ways, including coauthoring material, training research and community therapists, doing clinical supervision, watching hours and hours of therapy session tapes and defining and redefining terms for adherence measures, and reworking slides to come up with succinct but accurate phrases to convey the essence of complicated ideas. Consequently, Kelly knows DBT as few people do and has a unique ability to distill what is essential and to make it come alive with clinical examples. Moreover, she brings her own unique creativity and persona to the treatment, showing that DBT is anything but a rigid, follow-the-protocol-each-minute treatment.

Kelly's longtime meditation practice and study of the martial art aikido give her a deep understanding of the ways spiritual practices from Zen and contemplative prayer have influenced the development of DBT. In fact, when I watched her take her first-degree black-belt test in 1993, I realized that she was cultivating as an aikido practitioner the same deeply engaged compassion I encouraged as her DBT clinical supervisor, namely, the ability to meet difficult, even threatening, situations with a spirit of loving protection. Kelly has an embodied sense of dialectically balancing acceptance and change that shines through in her writing here.

It is with great joy and enthusiasm that I recommend Kelly's book to you. This book is a much-needed resource for any therapist learning and using DBT.

MARSHA M. LINEHAN, PhD

Preface

This book shows why, when, and how to use the principles and strategies of dialectical behavior therapy (DBT) in individual psychotherapy. Whereas Linehan's (1993a) original DBT book is a treatment manual, this book is a user's guide, full of clinical vignettes and step-by-step descriptions meant to make it easy for you to see how you can use DBT with your clients. Chapter 1 explains how individuals come to develop pervasive emotion dysregulation and subsequently how this may lead to problems that destroy clients' quality of life and derail their efforts to change in therapy. This chapter gives a complete overview of how DBT structures treatment to address this core problem of pervasive emotion dysregulation. In Chapter 2 I describe how to translate this general understanding of emotion dysregulation into the nitty-gritty steps of formulating cases and planning treatment for individual clients. I then turn to the three sets of core treatment strategies used in DBT to achieve clients' therapeutic goals: behavioral change strategies, validation strategies, and dialectical strategies. These are introduced in the first chapter and described in detail in Chapters 3, 4, and 5, respectively. Because pervasive emotion dysregulation leads to mood-dependent behavior and crises, the DBT therapist often must modify behavioral change strategies (i.e., the cognitive-behavioral procedures of skills training, exposure therapy, contingency management, and cognitive modification). These modifications are described fully in Chapter 3. Because clients with pervasive emotion dysregulation often experience change-oriented interventions as invalidating, DBT emphasizes the active, disciplined, and precise use of validation strategies. DBT's validation strategies have been better articulated by Linehan (1997) in the years since her original book was published; those updates, as well as extensive clinical examples that show how to validate as well as what (and what not) to validate, are covered in depth in

Chapter 4. In Chapter 5 I describe the dialectical stance and strategies that help the therapist completely accept the client and the moment as they are while simultaneously moving urgently for change. This third and final set of core strategies involves the ability to resist oversimplification and move beyond trade-offs to find genuinely workable blends of behavioral change and validation, reason and emotion, and acceptance and change. Chapter 6 brings the three sets of strategies together and illustrates how they are used in the context of the case formulation and hierarchy of treatment targets. Finally, Chapter 7 emphasizes the crucial importance and workings of the DBT peer consultation team—a community of therapists treating a community of clients while also applying DBT to themselves. The team strengthens therapists' skills and provides emotional support needed to meet the challenges that arise when clients face tremendous suffering and emotional pain. All clinical examples used in this book are fictional composites of many client–therapist dialogues intended to create the best teaching materials.

I have two hopes in writing this book. First, I have spent many years teaching and consulting to therapists as they learned to use DBT. Most therapists learned more quickly when we supplemented the treatment manual with easy-to-follow clinical examples of how DBT's principles and strategies are applied to specific cases. This book attempts to do just that—to provide extensive clinical examples illustrating the key moments in DBT in a way that I hope helps you more easily use DBT with your clients. Second, I hope to show how, even if you never use the entire package of comprehensive DBT, its principles nonetheless can provide you with a foundation in your work with clients who have complicated, severe, and chronic problems. The growing alphabet soup of treatment protocols and manuals can be overwhelming. DBT's principles and strategies offer a highly flexible heuristic framework that helps simplify complex clinical situations into a series of systematic, open-ended prompts to think or act. As Roger Martin (2009) puts it, "The beauty of heuristics is that they guide us toward a solution by way of organized exploration of the possibilities" (p. 12). Whatever your orientation, I hope I can show you how DBT's framework could help you systematically arrange elements of treatment into a comprehensive, individualized treatment plan.

Finally, my personal impetus for writing this book has been to try to pass along what I have so generously been given. I have had the unbelievable good fortune to work closely and for many years with DBT's treatment developer, Marsha M. Linehan, as well as with the amazingly talented and creative therapists who were DBT's early adopters. The collective work of this community of practitioners and the unmitigated honor of working with my own clients humble me and inspire me to match stride. May the effort here be of benefit to you.

Acknowledgments

Many teachers, colleagues, and loved ones have supported the writing of this book. John Gluck, Howard Delaney, and, especially, Michael Dougher's lab and his hilarious, demanding Radical Behaviorism course, mentored wide-ranging yet rigorous theoretical thinking. Neil Jacobson's insatiable intellectual productivity created tremendous opportunities for me to help develop and evaluate treatment and to write. Mark Greenberg's developmental psychopathology thought papers, Mavis Tsai and Robert Kohlenberg's close clinical supervision, and hundreds of hours coding the adherence to and competence of different psychotherapies shaped my views of how therapists help clients change. Cedar Koons, Meggan Moorhead, Clive Robbins, and Charley Huffine supported my early development as a clinical consultant. Most important, I joined Marsha M. Linehan's clinical practicum on dialectical behavior therapy (DBT) in 1989. Those were exciting days. Marsha carted in freshly mimeographed drafts of her treatment manuals and unapologetically recruited for us the most suicidal clients she could find. Our skill and camaraderie grew, until eventually the grad students in the practicum had difficulty finding supervisors who knew more than we did about helping highly suicidal individuals when Marsha left for her sabbatical. Marsha's generous years of weekly clinical supervision and of writing and teaching together led to our founding Behavioral Tech together in 1997, and now, ultimately, have come to fruition in this book. Marsha's courage, dedication, and personal sacrifice have shown me how a professional life of science and compassion can be a spiritual path as disciplined as any monastic tradition.

In 1988 I began studying aikido, a martial art that trains practitioners to meet conflict and violence with a spirit of loving protection. Aikido deeply informs my understanding of DBT. I am especially grateful for periods of resident study with Raso Hultgren Sensei and Tom Read Sensei. Their piercingly honest personal practice has shown me what it means to be a serious student.

Thanks to Jacqueline Persons and Kitty Moore for the opportunity to contribute to the Guides to Individualized Evidence-Based Treatment series and to Barbara Watkins for her developmental editing. Many thanks to colleagues who critiqued drafts, especially Jacqueline Persons, Niklas Toerneke, Carla Walton, and Scott Temple, and also to Michael Maslar and Elizabeth Simpson, who helped develop two of the clinical vignettes. Charlie Swenson's high-caliber teaching and writing inspired me, and his mentorship saw me through career challenges. Les Greenberg's work pervasively influenced my thinking about the importance of empathy and the view of the therapist as an emotion coach. Many thanks to Robert Butkiewicz for his support and to my writing group—Benjamin Schoendorff, Gareth Holman, Mavis Tsai, and Stig Helweg-Jørgensen—who carried me through the last leg of completing the manuscript.

All my love and gratitude go to Cindy Smith, psychiatrist and poet. Without her encouragement and editing, this book would not exist.

I thank with deep gratitude my extended kinship group of colleagues and clients. I have had the humbling honor of being witness and working partner as people faced unbearable vulnerability and emotional pain with integrity. In ways I still dimly understand, I have received as much or more than I have given. To walk with kindred spirits whom I so greatly admire has been a gift of immeasurable value.

Thanks, finally, to Claire and Tom Winter for their love and support over the many years this book has occupied our lives.

Contents

DOING DIALECTICAL BEHAVIOR THERAPY

ONE

Tools for Tough Circumstances

If you've picked up this book, it's likely that the grim statistics on treatment failure come as no surprise to you. As therapists, we can all recall cases in which, despite our best efforts, our usual ways of working failed our clients. When clients come to us prone to emotion dysregulation, with multiple, serious, chronic problems, and with a history of failed therapy relationships, we know the odds are against us.

"It doesn't matter what I do, nothing changes."

Marie is in her mid-20s. She comes to her third session of individual therapy agitated and tells her therapist that she has "completely lost it" at work. She's going to be fired, and that means she will be evicted when she can't pay the rent. When the therapist asks what happened, Marie angrily jerks her body, kicking the coffee table in the process. It's not clear if she meant to kick the table or if it was an accident, but she flushes red from head to toe, becomes mute, and curls up in the chair. She begins to bang her head against the armrest. This derails any help the therapist might have offered regarding the crisis at work, and the way she acts in therapy creates a new situation about which Marie will feel shame. As the therapist gets Marie to stop banging her head, Marie says quietly, "I just need to end this." Given Marie's history of near-lethal suicide attempts, the therapist now must manage to assess imminent suicide risk with a mostly mute, overwhelmed, and soon-to-be-homeless client.

If you met Mark at a party, you'd assume he worked in a funky, successful high-tech firm. You'd never guess he barely scrapes by on temp work as a software programmer. His life has become more and more restricted by anxiety and brief manic episodes that are followed by crashes into self-loathing. For months, he stays trashed with marijuana, alcohol, and anti-anxiety medication. He sleeps 18 hours a day, leaving his house only to get food. After 15 years of working with many therapists, he's not sure whether to blame them or himself that his life remains miserable.

For clients like Marie and Mark, exquisite vulnerability to emotions and intense emotional pain defeat a quality life. Unrelenting misery makes thoughts of suicide or nonsuicidal self-injury among the few things that offer relief. Repeated treatment failures make therapy itself evoke intense hopelessness.

Treatment decisions we make in such circumstances are extremely complicated. When we focus on how the client needs to change, the client panics because such efforts have often failed in the past. It also triggers either anger or shame at the implication that change is possible: you, the therapist, don't have a clue about how impossible change actually is, or else you believe, as others have, that the problem is the client's poor motivation or personality flaws. When, in response, we drop a change orientation and instead focus on accepting vulnerability and limitations, this too sets off panic in the client, especially despair that things will never change. Out of desperation, your client may reject the help that you offer and demand help that you cannot give. Suicide attempts, threats of suicide, and the anger directed at us are stressful. Our own emotions, confusion, or skills deficits complicate matters further, leading us to expect change beyond the client's capability and to fail to offer sufficient warmth, flexibility, or resourcefulness when needed. The non-stop effort of striking the right balance—accepting the client's true vulnerability while also insisting on change—wears us down. It might as easily have been us, as therapists, saying, "I can't take this. It doesn't matter what I do—nothing changes."

Dialectical behavior therapy, or DBT (Linehan, 1993a), evolved to help therapists and clients in exactly these circumstances, and a growing number of randomized clinical trials support its efficacy (see review by Lynch, Trost, Salsman, & Linehan, 2006). When clients have complicated, severe, chronic problems and multiple treatment providers, when misery makes suicide seem the client's only option, DBT helps therapists find order amid chaos. As a comprehensive outpatient treatment package, DBT structures the treatment environment into weekly individual therapy, weekly group skills training, telephone coaching, and a peer consultation team of DBT therapists. Within that environment, DBT consists of a hierarchy of treatment priorities and core strategies for addressing those priorities. These features offer systematic guidelines for clinical decision making that help therapists treat life-threatening and therapy-interfering behaviors as well as their own emotional reactions. This book presents how DBT is conducted from the perspective of the individual therapist, illustrating why, when, and how to use DBT's tools to achieve therapeutic progress.

In the same way that protocols and procedures in an emergency room allow coordinated action, comprehensive DBT is essential for clients with suicidal crises like Marie. In cases like Mark's, you may not need the full model yet DBT's basic theories, hierarchy of priorities, and treatment strategies remain relevant. For this reason, I have organized this book to help clinicians in both sets of circumstances. You can adopt only those elements of DBT most likely to be helpful to you and your clients while also coming to understand the full therapeutic framework of DBT as a package so that you can structure the treatment environment and your clinical decision making when needed.

This book recognizes that the science on which DBT draws is constantly evolving: new data from research on the development and evaluation of DBT as well as the psychopathology and disorders it is used to treat must be continually integrated in order to offer our patients the best possible clinical care. Linehan (1993a) developed DBT first as a treatment for chronic suicidal behavior, and then subsequently for borderline personality disorder (BPD). However, the very diagnosis of BPD has undergone extensive revision and will likely continue to do so. As new data emerge, we can expect the components of DBT to change as well as the kinds of clients for whom it is indicated. To date, for example, published randomized controlled trials conducted by different research teams support the efficacy of DBT across a wide variety of behavioral problems, including suicide attempts and self-injurious behaviors (Koons et al., 2001; Linehan, Armstrong, Suarez, Allmon, & Heard, 1991; Linehan, Heard, & Armstrong, 1993; Linehan, Comtois, Murray, et al., 2006; van den Bosch, Koeter, Stijnen, Verheul, & van den Brink, 2005; Verheul et al., 2003), substance abuse (Linehan et al., 1999, 2002), bulimia (Safer, Telch, & Agras, 2001), binge eating (Telch, Agras, & Linehan, 2001), and depression in the elderly (Lynch, Morse, Mendelson, & Robins, 2003; Lynch et al., 2007). This makes it important to realize that DBT is not only indicated for chronically suicidal behavior and BPD. DBT's set of principles and protocols can be applied more broadly to arrange cognitive-behavioral and other theoretically compatible strategies to treat disorders characterized by pervasive emotion dysregulation. An important aim of this book, therefore, is to make it easy for you to flexibly use DBT's comprehensive package or its components to keep up to date with the latest research findings.

A first step in helping you use DBT flexibly is understanding the core problem of clients like Marie and Mark: pervasive emotion dysregulation. Linehan's biosocial theory, described next in this chapter, explains how this core problem can lead to such diverse and difficult secondary problems. DBT's treatment components follow from an understanding of pervasive emotion dysregulation and its impact. These components are described in the second half of this chapter. Key among them is the way that client problems are ranked according to the threat they pose to a reasonable quality of life. This hierarchy of treatment goals and targets guides case formulation (covered in detail Chapter 2) and in-session clinical decision making. The therapist uses it to give the most important tasks priority over the less important. Three sets of core treatment strategies are then used to move the client toward therapeutic goals. The core strategy sets—behavioral change strategies, validation strategies, and dialectical strategies—are first introduced in this chapter and then described in detail in Chapters 3, 4, and 5, respectively. Chapter 6 brings the three sets of strategies together, illustrating how they are used in the context of the case formulation and hierarchy of treatment targets. Finally, Chapter 7 emphasizes the crucial importance and workings of the DBT peer consultation team—a requirement of comprehensive DBT. The consultation team is a community of therapists treating a community of patients while also applying DBT to themselves. The team strengthens therapists' skills and provides emotional support needed to meet the challenges that arise when clients face tremendous suffering and emotional pain. Understanding DBT starts with understanding this core problem—pervasive emotion dysregulation.

THE CORE PROBLEM
OF PERVASIVE EMOTION DYSREGULATION

Linehan explained the etiology and maintenance of BPD with a biosocial theory of emotion dysregulation. DBT has since been adapted for use across disorders and patient populations (e.g., substance abuse, bulimia, and antisocial and other personality disorders), but the biosocial theory has remained central (see Crowell, Beauchaine, & Linehan, 2009, for a recent review). It proposes that pervasive emotion dysregulation arises from the combination of vulnerable biology and invalidating social environments. Emotion dysregulation is the inability, despite one's best efforts, to change or regulate emotional cues, experiences, actions, verbal responses, and/ or nonverbal expressions under normative conditions. Pervasive emotion dysregulation is when this inability to regulate emotions occurs across a wide range of emotions, problems, and situational contexts. (Linehan, Bohus, & Lynch, 2007). Such difficulties with dysregulation lead to maladaptive behaviors (e.g., suicidal behavior, purging, abusing substances), because these behaviors function to regulate emotions or are a consequence of failed emotion regulation.

Biosocial Theory: The Impact of Vulnerable Biology and Invalidating Social Environment

Vulnerable Biology and Its Consequences

Linehan hypothesized that three biologically based characteristics contribute to an individual's vulnerability. First, people prone to emotion dysregulation react immediately and at low thresholds (high sensitivity). Second, they experience and express emotion intensely (high reactivity), and this high arousal dysregulates cognitive processes too. Third, they experience a long-lasting arousal (slow return to baseline). In fact, the data do suggest that those who meet the criteria for BPD experience more frequent, more intense, and longer-lasting aversive states (Stiglmayr et al., 2005) and that biological vulnerability may contribute to difficulties regulating emotion (e.g., Juengling et al., 2003; Ebner-Priemer et al., 2005).

Consider the impact of such biological vulnerability. Difficulty regulating emotion means difficulty regulating most areas of one's life: most of what we do and who we are depends on mood stability and adequate emotion regulation. The same action may feel easy or hard depending on our mood. Take the common experience of schmoozing with strangers at a cocktail party. In a great mood, you breeze right up to chat with the most interesting person in the room; in a vulnerable, insecure mood, you cling to the wall, barely making eye contact. You put off a dreaded task for months. Later, in the right mood—voilà—you tackle it in an afternoon. Those of us who can regulate emotion without much effort take this ability for granted. We occasionally have bouts of mood-dependent behavior, but for the most part we muddle through.

Imagine, however, that due to biological vulnerability your emotions instead vary wildly. You can't predict what mood you'll be in. If your behavior varies wildly at social gatherings based on your mood, are you a shy person or an outgoing person? If you can manage responsibilities when you're "together enough" emotionally, does that make you irresponsible and lazy when you can't manage? Are you cut out for school or a certain type of work? How can you tell when your ability to perform seems largely beyond your control and dependent on your emotional state? The impact of this unpredictable variability affects all areas of life. Like living in a nightmare, your efforts have no effect or go terribly wrong. This biological vulnerability is exacerbated, and in some cases even created, by transactions between the emotionally vulnerable person and a social environment that is pervasively invalidating.

Invalidating Social Environment and Its Consequences

Think first about emotional development in an optimally validating environment. Emotion evolves as a rapid, whole-body response: our physiology, perception, actions, and cognitive processes coherently fire together, orienting and organizing adaptation to continual changes in the environment and in our bodies. We hear an unexpected noise, and immediately emotion fires, orienting us so we're prepared. In healthy emotional development, caregivers respond to a child in ways that strengthen the links between environmental cues, primary emotions, and socially appropriate emotional expression while weakening the links for socially inappropriate expression. Our caregivers' responses validate what is effective, appropriate, and makes sense about our responses and invalidate that which is ineffective, inappropriate, and does not make sense. For example, based on these processes of acculturation, we learn to interpret certain noises as cues for interest or fear, and learn to modulate how we express what we feel. Others' validating responses teach us to use emotion to understand what is happening within and outside our skin as a moment-to-moment readout of our own state and our needs with respect to the environment. In an optimal environment, caregivers provide contingent, appropriate soothing for strong emotions. They strengthen and help the individual refine the naturally adaptive, organizing, and communicative functions of emotions.

None of us get the perfectly optimal environment, of course. Even the best parents are tired; they're stressed. They are themselves habitually anxious, angry, or depressed. From these compromised states, they punish or minimize valid expression of primary emotions. We consequently learn more or less dysfunctional ways of expressing and making sense of our emotions. Bigger problems arise, however, when caregivers *consistently* and *persistently* fail to respond as needed to primary emotion and its expression. Pervasive invalidation occurs when, more often than not, caregivers treat our valid primary responses as incorrect, inaccurate, inappropriate, pathological, or not to be taken seriously. Primary responses of interest are persistently squelched or mocked; normal needs for soothing are regularly neglected or shamed; honest motives consistently doubted and misinterpreted. The person therefore learns to avoid, interrupt, and control his or her own natural inclinations and primary emotional responses. Like a creature in a chamber with an electrified grid for the floor, he or she learns to avoid any step that results in pain and invalidation.

For example, say that in contrast to my well-regulated siblings, I express more need for affection or express emotions longer and more intensely than fits my caregiver's tolerance. This repeatedly provokes impatience and scorn (invalidation). Eventually I attempt to inhibit my behavior, perhaps by learning to inhibit both overt behaviors that express my need for affection and maybe even my private experience of needing it. In pervasively invalidating environments, fear conditioning takes place—we not only avoid the electric grid of invalidation, but also avoid any experience of the private events (thoughts, sensations, or emotions) which might lead anywhere near the grid. We become extremely sensitized to all cues that might bring on the painful zap of invalidation. We become phobic of our own valid, natural responses. Histories of pervasive invalidation leave people not only hypersensitive to others' invalidation, but sensitive to any response of their own, valid or not, that might prompt others to invalidate them. Responding naturally is often as evocative as dropping a spider in the lap of someone with a spider phobia.

In Linehan's theory, different combinations of biological vulnerability and social invalidation can result in fairly similar experiences. People may also travel different developmental routes yet end up with the same difficulties. For those with a high biological vulnerability to emotion dysregulation, even a "normal" level of invalidation may be sufficient to create serious problems. Like those with attention deficits, they face enormous but often hard-to-perceive difficulties. For example, if one child with normal attentional processes and one with attention-deficit/hyperactivity disorder (ADHD) are playing a board game and getting too rowdy, a stern "Settle down in there!" from an adult in the kitchen is enough for the kid with normal attention capabilities to comply. But the kid with ADHD may need the adult to come in and provide step-by-step coaching: "No. It's not your turn. Give the dice to Joey. Sweetie, look at me. Set the dice down. Thanks. OK, now watch. It's Joey's turn. No, put your hands in your lap. That's it. Let's see, he got a five . . ." (and so forth). Over time and with practice, such coaching turns into self-regulation. The same active coaching approach is also needed to help those trying to manage pervasive emotion dysregulation. As with attention dysregulation, additional guidance and structure are required to develop self-regulation of emotion. Few parents know how to provide such help; most parents can be overwhelmed by the needs of a highly vulnerable child. Consequently, such emotionally vulnerable children seldom learn effective strategies to manage their overwhelming emotional experience. DBT targets these deficits and explicitly teaches the skills required to regulate emotion.

Other people begin life with very little biological vulnerability, but experience such extreme and persistent invalidation over time that they develop problems regulating emotion. Childhood sexual abuse is a prototypical invalidating environment related to BPD (Wagner & Linehan, 1997, 2006). However, not all individuals who meet BPD criteria report histories of sexual abuse, and not all victims of childhood sexual abuse develop

BPD. It remains unclear how to account for individual differences (e.g., see Rosenthal, Cheavens, Lejuez, & Lynch, 2005, for one line of research beginning to piece together the mediational factors between BPD symptoms and childhood sexual abuse). Linehan (1993a) has therefore argued that it is the experience of pervasive invalidation that is causal rather than any one specific type of trauma. Such histories leave people extremely sensitized to invalidation.

The difficulties I've described so far follow from the core problem of emotion dysregulation. When the environment poorly fits our needs, whether due to biological vulnerability or pervasive invalidation, we learn a range of problematic emotion regulation strategies. When our normative experience and expression of emotion elicits discomfort in others who then withdraw and criticize rather than help and support us, we learn that who we are and how we are evokes interpersonal rejection. We thereby learn to avoid our valid primary responses and instead develop patterns of blunting, masking, and/or distorting our experience and expression of emotions. Avoidance may be subtle: we protect ourselves when we sense a slight inattention in our friend as we speak by changing what we were going to say to a less risky self-disclosure; without awareness we rapidly escape a vulnerable first flash of sadness or shame by feeling irritated. Avoidance may be obvious, full-out escape: our emotional state is so aversive that we either involuntarily escape it by dissociating or find desperate methods such as intentional self-injury to end emotional pain. While such learning processes affect us all, those prone to emotion dysregulation experience more pervasive social invalidation and come to alternate between strategies that overregulate and underregulate emotion and its expression. These problematic behavioral patterns wreak havoc in clients' lives and in therapy and are discussed next.

Dialectical Dilemmas: Secondary Behavioral Patterns

Managing emotion vulnerability and ongoing invalidation often strands the client in a dilemma between overregulating and underegulating emotional experience and expression. Linehan called these patterns "dialectical dilemmas" because an essential idea of "dialectics" is that any one position contains its own antithesis or opposite position. The client's inevitable failures to regulate emotion lead to increased invalidation ("Why are you so sensitive?," "You're crazy!," or "Get over it!"), which in turn leads to redoubled efforts to self-regulate in order to avoid further invalidation. At the other extreme, clients may escalate expression as they try to communicate why their responses *are* valid ("I'm not crazy! You don't understand!"). Over time, common behavioral patterns develop as clients attempt to resolve the dilemmas inherent in pervasive emotion dysregulation. Through clinical observation, Linehan characterized three patterns in which clients flipped from underregulated states in which the client is overwhelmed by emotional experience to overregulated states with rapid avoidance of emotional experience.

Emotion Vulnerability and Self-Invalidation

Biological vulnerability and a history of pervasive invalidation create exquisite sensitivity. The slightest cue can set off emotional pain, the equivalent of touching third-degree burns. Because the individual cannot control the onset and offset of events that trigger emotional responses, the person can become desperate for anything that will make the pain end. For many, it's as if their physical body cannot withstand the forces raging through it. Even dysregulation of positive emotions creates pain. For example, a client reported, "I got so excited when I saw my friends, I couldn't stand it. I laughed too loud, talked too much—everything I did was too big for them." "Emotion vulnerability" refers not only to the exquisite sensitivity but further to the consequences of living as a person who is exquisitely sensitive. Unavoidable day-to-day experiences trigger intense emotional pain to the point where having emotions can become traumatic: people in this situation cannot tell when they will be undone by emotions. Performance becomes totally unpredictable because it is tied to emotional states the person is unable to control. This unpredictability foils personal and interpersonal expectations leading the client and others to feel frustrated and disillusioned. The person despairs because she experiences her emotional sensitivity as biological, as part of her temperament, and therefore as something that will never change. The client finds herself trapped in a nightmare of dyscontrol. Life is a continual fight to endure a typical day's events. Suicide may seem the only way to prevent future excruciating suffering. Suicide can also be a final communication to unsympathetic others.

For exquisitely sensitive people, nearly any therapeutic movement evokes emotional pain, much as debridement does in the treatment of serious burns. Sensitivity to criticism makes it painful to receive needed feedback. As we saw in the case of Marie at the beginning of this chapter, in-session emotion dysregulation (dissociation, panic, intense anger) interrupts therapeutic tasks. The generalization of changes and plans made in session goes awry due to emotion dysregulation in daily life. Therapy itself may be traumatic because the client cannot regulate the emotion evoked in therapy. Clients often feel humiliated by their helplessness in the face of overwhelming emotion. Understanding emotion vulnerability means the therapist must understand and reckon with the intense pain involved in living without "emotional skin."

People learn to respond to their ongoing vulnerability to emotion dysregulation by invalidating themselves, just as others have done. Self-invalidation takes at least two forms. In the first, the person judges dysregulation harshly ("I shouldn't be this way"). Here, the person attempts to control and avoid natural primary responses. When this fails, the person turns against the self with self-blame and self-hatred. Intentional self-injury may be used to punish oneself for failure. In the second, the person may deny and ignore the vulnerability to dysregulation ("I am *not* this way"), block emotional experience, and hold unrealistically high or perfectionistic expectations. In doing so, the person minimizes the difficulty of solving life problems and fails to recognize more help is needed. This pattern often defeats attempts to change as the person won't tolerate the trial-and-error learning needed to acquire self-management strategies.

Active Passivity and Apparent Competence

Over time, people learn to respond passively when they are left with problems that are beyond their capability while the difficulties of solving them are minimized. At times, remaining passive activates others. Seeing a vulnerable-looking woman staring helplessly at a flat tire on the side of the road in a bad neighborhood might prompt someone to stop to help. If help doesn't arrive, she might express more distress—frantically checking her watch and beginning to cry. Active passivity is the tendency to respond to problems passively in the face of insufficient help while communicating distress in ways that activate others.

For example, Mark, who we met at the start of this chapter, barely scrapes by as a software programmer because his perfectionism, procrastination, and moodiness have led to many missed deadlines—so many that his latest employer did not renew his contract. Devastated and ashamed, he hides out, refusing to answer calls and putting his mail into a drawer unopened. When his landlord's patience ends, he asks Mark to move out. Instead of searching for a new place to live, Mark spends the day in bed and is silent during therapy despite all efforts by the therapist to encourage active problem solving. Mark experiences himself as unable to do what is necessary and he actually is unable to act without more help. If he had just broken a leg, help might be forthcoming. However, without observable deficits, others view him as lazy. When he asks others for help he is ineffective—others experience him as demanding and whiney. Mark's experience, however, is that the situation is hopeless no matter what he does. From the therapist's perspective, the situation worsens into a crisis that could easily be solved if Mark would cope actively (e.g., check Craigslist to find another place). When this pattern of active passivity is habitual, it increases life stress as problems go unsolved; it alienates helpers; and it makes suicide one of the few means of communicating that more help is needed.

Apparent competence is deadly. At one moment the client appears able to cope and then (unexpectedly to the observer) at other times it's as if the competency did not exist. Clients have learned to "appear competent" that is, to hide emotion and vulnerability so that observers see very little expressed emotion. Often clients may verbalize negative emotions but nonverbally convey little, if any, distress. Yet their internal experience is that they have just screamed their distress—they have become so sensitized to their own expression that simply saying anything at all feels naked and raw. When verbal and nonverbal expressions of emotion are incongruous, we all default to believing that the nonverbal is the more accurate expression. Therapists (and others in the client's life) are likely in these instances to misread. If a client says to you, "That really bothered me" in a matter-of-fact voice, it is easy to think that he or she is basically OK and miss the actual experience of extreme but unexpressed distress. A second misreading can come from the typical assumption that behaviors generalize (i.e., if I am friendly and outgoing at one party, I will be friendly and outgoing at the next party). However, as described above, mood influences how difficult or easy it is to perform many behaviors. When the core problem is emotion dysregulation, clients have little control of their emotional state and therefore little control over their behavioral capabilities. This will produce variable and conditional competence across settings and over time. Yet observers (and the client herself) will expect continuity and be repeatedly surprised when a competency fails to generalize as it might with more emotionally regulated people. Because others misread, they inadvertently create an invalidating environment, failing to help because they cannot see the distress. In the worst cases, others interpret the absence of expected competence as manipulation and become less willing to help.

Unrelenting Crisis and Inhibited Grieving

Unrelenting crisis refers to a self-perpetuating pattern in which a person both creates and is controlled by incessant aversive events. An emotionally vulnerable person may impulsively act to decrease distress; this can inadvertently increase problems that quickly snowball into worse problems. For example, Marie "lost it" at work, and is going to be fired which in turn can lead to eviction from her apartment. Another client yells in anger at a case worker and impulsively ends an interview. This means that the needed housing application is not completed. When another appointment cannot be scheduled, the client ends up in a homeless shelter. Residing in a homeless shelter then exposes the client to a host of cues that remind her of a past rape, setting off daily flashbacks and panic attacks. Such unrelenting crises can dominate therapy to such an extent that it is difficult to make progress.

Inhibited grieving is an involuntary, automatic avoidance of painful emotional experiences, an inhibition of the natural unfolding of emotional responding. The tragedies that some of our clients have endured have been shattering. They may inhibit grief associated with childhood trauma or revictimization as an adult, or grief evoked by current losses that are the consequence of maladaptive coping or inordinately bad luck. To stop the emotional pain, they avoid and escape which inadvertently increases sensitization to emotion cues and reactions. Some clients constantly experience loss, start the mourning process, automatically inhibit the process by avoiding or distracting from relevant cues, reenter the process, and cycle through contact with the cue and escape, over and again. The individual never fully experiences, integrates, or resolves reactions to painful events.

The three behavioral patterns described above are the developmental fallout from the toxic combination of biological vulnerability and social invalidation. While all of us develop habitual, somewhat problematic reactions to our own emotional pain, these three patterns wreak havoc. Daily life and therapy in particular offer a gauntlet of evocative cues: the client's own behaviors or others' behaviors may prompt dysregulation. These secondary responses to dysregulation, in which the client oscillates from under- to overregulating emotion, create further serious problems. Consequently, the behavioral patterns themselves become treatment targets in DBT.

In summary, then, the first key component of DBT is the biosocial theory of disorder. It proposes that (1) problematic or disordered behavior, particularly extremely dysfunctional behaviors, may be a consequence of emotion dysregulation or an effort to re-regulate emotion; (2) invalidation plays a role in maintenance of current difficulties regulating emotion; and (3) common patterns subsequently develop as a person struggles to regulate emotion and deal with invalidation; these patterns become problems that themselves must be treated. DBT's overarching treatment rationale therefore is to teach and support emotion regulation and to reinstate the natural organizing and communicative functions of emotion.

HOW DBT TREATS
PERVASIVE EMOTION DYSREGULATION

DBT treats pervasive emotion dysregulation and the subsequent common patterns that develop as the individual copes with pervasive emotion dysregulation with the following: a combination of core treatment strategies—change, acceptance, and dialectical strategies—summarized in Table 1.1 and a framework of guidelines that structures the treatment environment and prioritizes treatment goals and targets according to the extent of the client's disorder.

Core Treatment Strategies

Change Strategies

DBT's first set of core strategies focus on change, weaving together behavioral principles and protocols from cognitive-behavioral and other theoretically compatible strategies to treat pervasive emotion dysregulation. Behavioral chain analysis—a form of functional analysis—is used to identify the variables that control specific instances of targeted problems such as self-injury. DBT case formulation is based on the functional patterns that emerge from these chain analyses. Treatment plans address what needs to go differently in the behavioral chain so that the client does not engage in the problem behavior. Some clients, like Mark introduced earlier in this chapter, lack basic capabilities needed to regulate emotion and, therefore, part of DBT's solution is to teach skills to remedy these deficits. Skills training is discussed later in this chapter.

But learning new skills is not always enough. For example, the capabilities Mark does have are often disrupted by conditioned emotional responses, problematic contingencies and dysfunctional cognitive processes. Therefore, DBT's change strategies include not only skills training but also three other groups of cognitive-behavioral procedures: exposure therapy, contingency management, and cognitive modification. However, because pervasive dysregulation leads to mood-dependent behavior and crises, the DBT therapist must often modify these standard cognitive-behavioral therapy (CBT) interventions to be successful. These modifications are described fully in Chapter 3. Change strategies also include techniques for increasing client motivation and commitment to change. These commitment strategies include pros and cons, devil's advocate, shaping, and others listed in Table 1.1. Behavioral expertise is required in DBT. A lack of behavioral expertise is a genuine barrier to the therapist who wishes to work from a DBT framework.

Validation Strategies

DBT's second core set of strategies, validation, emphasizes acceptance. For example, Mark's history has left him exquisitely sensitive to invalidation. This sensitivity led to him losing his job: his boss's requests for change

TABLE 1.1. DBT Core Strategies at a Glance

Behavioral change strategies (change-oriented)

- Behavioral chain analysis
- Task analyses
- Solution analyses
- Skills training (see Table 1.2)
- Self-monitoring: the DBT diary card
- Exposure
- Contingency management
- Cognitive modification
- Didactic strategies (psychoeducation)
- Orienting
- Commitment strategies
  - Pros and cons
  - Foot-in-the-door
  - Door-in-the-face
  - Freedom to choose; absence of alternatives
  - Linking prior commitments to current commitments
  - Devil's advocate
  - Shaping

Validation strategies (acceptance-oriented)

- Empathy + communicating client's perspective is valid in some way
  - Level 1: Listen with complete awareness; be awake
  - Level 2: Accurately reflect the client's communication
  - Level 3: Articulate unverbalized emotions, thoughts, or behavior patterns
  - Level 4: Communicate how behavior makes sense in terms of past circumstances
  - Level 5: Communicate how behavior makes sense in current circumstances
  - Level 6: Be radically genuine

Dialectical strategies

- Dialectical assumptions and dialectical stance
- Dialectical balancing
  - Change and validation strategies
  - Stylistic strategies: Reciprocal and irreverent
  - Case management strategies: Consultation to the client and environmental intervention
- Specific dialectical strategies
  - Dialectical assessment
  - Entering the paradox
  - Metaphor
  - Devil's advocate
  - Extending
  - Activating wise mind
  - Making lemonade
  - Allowing natural change

overwhelmed him and his prior therapist's attempts to help him change appropriately in response to the poor performance evaluations felt excruciating to him. Much of Mark's responding was ineffective and needed to change, but for clients like Mark, change interventions feel intolerable. Validation strategies therefore become crucial. Validation comes from the client-centered tradition (Linehan 1997b; see also the excellent book *Empathy Reconsidered*, by Bohart & Greenberg, 1997). DBT defines validation as empathy plus the communication that the client's perspective is valid in some way. With empathy, you accurately understand the world from the client's perspective; with validation you also actively communicate that the client's perspective makes sense.

It might be tempting to lump validation with "facilitative conditions" or "common factors," or to relegate it to "the sugar that helps the medicine go down," as if to coax the client to engage in the "real thing," of change-oriented strategies. However, validation, *in itself*, can produce powerful change when it is active, disciplined, and precise. Used genuinely and with skill, it reduces physiological arousal that is a normal effect of invalidation and it can cue more adaptive emotions to fire. Skill in the use of validation strategies centers on what (and what not) to validate as well as how to validate. Linehan (1997b) listed six levels of validation as shown in Table 1.1 and she advised therapists to validate at the highest possible level. Validation strategies are covered in depth in Chapter 4.

Dialectical Strategies

The tension between the need to accept clients' true vulnerabilities and yet encourage them to make necessary change is a constant dilemma for the therapist and often the root of therapeutic impasse. To navigate, therapists take a dialectical stance and use dialectical strategies. Dialectics is both a view about the nature of reality and a method of persuasion. In both, an essential idea is that any one position contains its antithesis or opposite position. Progress comes from the resolution of the two opposing positions into a synthesis. In other words, the way forward is to simultaneously accept the client *and* push for change. Polarization is natural and expected. Therapeutic movement happens by keeping both ends of a polarity in play. In DBT, therapeutic impasse signals the need to explore both poles of the dialectical tension.

Dialectical strategies provide the practical means for both the therapist and the client to retain flexibility amid conflicting and even contradictory "truths." For example, in Mark's past therapies, when the therapist pushed too hard for change, Mark would no show for the next session. When the therapist dropped a change focus, accepting Mark's vulnerabilities, he became despairing and highly critical of the therapist's ineffectiveness—then also failed to show for appointments. This tension between acceptance of vulnerability and need for change is even more pronounced with clients like Marie. Marie and her therapist made it through the tough session that started this chapter. By the session's end, they'd generated a crisis plan to help Marie avert a suicide attempt. Although Marie left the office in better shape, the therapist feared more crisis behavior on the part of his client. Later that afternoon, Marie saw her pharmacotherapist. Not wanting to be dishonest, Marie described to him how intensely she wished she were dead; she explained that she liked her new therapist but was not sure she could follow through on the crisis plan they created; she's terrified about her ability to control her suicidal behavior. The pharmacotherapist decided that Marie needed to be hospitalized. He sent her directly to the nearest emergency room for evaluation. The next morning, instead of the expected check-in call from Marie, the individual therapist arrived to a message from the charge nurse at the local state hospital: between leaving her pharmacotherapist's office and reaching the emergency room, Marie took an overdose and then was involuntarily committed for 72 hours' observation.

Taking a dialectical perspective means one understands that suicidal clients like Marie often *simultaneously* want to live and want to die. Saying aloud to her therapist, "I want to die" rather than killing herself in secrecy contains within it the opposite position of "I want to live." This doesn't mean wanting to live is "more true" than wanting to die: she genuinely does not want to live her life. Nor does the low lethality of her suicide attempt mean that she really did not want to die. It's not even that she alternates between the two—she simultaneously holds both opposing positions. The client sees suicide as the only option out of an unbearable life. Rather than become polarized, in a dialectical approach the therapist agrees that the client's life is unbearable and that the client needs a way out, and offers another route, using therapy to build a life that is genuinely worth living. As will be described in more detail in Chapter 5, adopting a dialectical stance means embracing a worldview in which you can hold the position of completely accepting the client and moment as they are while simultaneously moving urgently for change. This third and final set of core strategies involves the ability to resist oversimplification and move beyond trade-offs to find genuinely workable blends of problem solving and validation, reason and emotion, and acceptance and change.

Clients who have experienced repeated suicidal crises and psychiatric hospitalizations often face a complicated web of interconnected problems. In these complicated, high-risk circumstances, more is needed than the biosocial theory and core strategies described so far. For example, one client's hospitalizations were prompted by invalidating interactions with minimally trained, overworked staff in her residential placement. The only way the client was able to get staff attention and help was through expressing extreme emotion and out-of-control behavior. In her case, providing crisis management as a stopgap to reduce acute problems could end up dominating therapy to such an extent that efficient, effective treatment becomes unlikely. Perhaps training the staff to better respond might be a better long-term solution. However, because staff turnover was sky high, whoever was trained would likely be gone within the month. Instead, it may be more efficient to train the client until her skills are so robust that she could regulate emotion even in the face of staff invalidation. But that would take time and, in truth, it would be an incredible challenge for anyone to regulate emotion in such a chaotic living situation. It's clear that without significant changes, leaving her in the residential setting will be a recipe for continued crises and psychiatric hospitalizations, yet making the needed changes within the setting appears daunting if not improbable.

Perhaps a better option would be to encourage her to move out of the residential setting. Yet without the structured activity of a residential placement, she will go downhill into inactivity and rumination. Her parents will panic at the thought that they will have to pick up the pieces if she is not living in a structured environment and it's not clear they would financially support such a move (or the therapist who proposes it!). For successful social activity outside a structured environment, she'd need friendships, which would require better social skills than she has. This in turn would actually require that she could tolerate your corrective feedback of her social skills and get through a group skills training session without becoming so dysregulated that she storms out of the room when invalidated.

Where to begin? Horst Rittel's term "wicked problems" (Rittel & Webber, 1973) captures the way that complex interdependencies among problems make it difficult even to conceptualize how to solve one aspect of the problem without creating another problem. With wicked problems, there are so many complicated relationships and dependencies among problems that beginning to work on one often leads to work on several others.

DBT's answer to wicked problems is to add structure. DBT structures the treatment environment according to the client's level of disorder. The more disordered the client's behavior, the more services are needed and the more comprehensive the treatment. Furthermore, with clients who have repeated suicidal crises like Marie, DBT adopts a framework of protocols and procedures that structure the therapist's clinical decision making and work in much the same way protocols and procedures in an emergency room allow coordinated action amid urgency and uncertainty.

Structuring the Treatment Environment

Standard comprehensive DBT as it has been manualized and researched is structured to provide all the treatment that a highly disordered client needs in order to achieve an acceptable quality of life. Comprehensive treatment for highly disordered clients, from this viewpoint, requires that treatment accomplish five functions that follow from the impact of pervasive emotional dysregulation described earlier. These are:

1. Enhance client capabilities. People with pervasive emotion dysregulation usually lack capabilities for effectively regulating emotion; they need to learn new skills and sometimes receive pharmacotherapy to enhance their capabilities.
2. Improve client motivation to change. As discussed earlier, clients often feel hopeless about change and have learned to be passive in the face of problems; they need help in becoming motivated to learn and then use new responses.
3. Ensure that new client capabilities generalize to the natural environment. Because emotion dysregulation keeps newly learned responses from readily generalizing, generalization to different settings and circumstances must be directly addressed.
4. Enhance therapist capabilities and motivation to treat clients effectively. Client emotion dysregulation, unrelenting crises, and suicidal behaviors wear down therapists' motivation and often stretch their skills to the limit. Therefore, therapists need support, motivation, and ways to increase their own skills.
5. Structure the environment in the ways essential to support client and therapist capabilities (Linehan, 1996, 1997a; Linehan et al., 1999). Particularly when emotional intensity and crises are an expected part of the work, everyone must know their role and what to do and what not to do to provide a clear, coherent, and well-organized approach. When treatment fails, it is often because it has failed to function in one or more of these ways; as a result, client and/or therapist needs were not met.

In standard comprehensive DBT, the above functions are spread among various modes of service delivery. Table 1.2 summarizes the above treatment functions along with examples of service modes. For example, clients in comprehensive treatment may receive weekly individual psychotherapy, weekly group skills training, telephone coaching of skills, and therapists participate in weekly or biweekly meetings of a DBT peer consultation team. The client and the individual therapist form the core of the treatment team, and they then engage other providers and loved ones

TABLE 1.2. Functions and Treatment Modes of Comprehensive DBT

Functions	Modes
Enhancing clients' capabilities: Helping clients acquire responses for effective performance	Skills training (individual or group), pharmacotherapy, psychoeducation
Improving motivation: Strengthening clinical progress and helping reduce factors that inhibit and/or interfere with progress (e.g., emotions, cognitions, overt behavior, environmental factors)	Individual psychotherapy, milieu treatment
Ensuring generalization: Transferring skillful response repertoire from therapy to clients' natural environment and helping integrate skillful responses within the changing natural environment	Skills coaching, milieu treatment, therapeutic communities, *in vivo* interventions, review of session tapes, involvement of family/friends
Enhancing therapists' skills and motivations: Acquiring, integrating, and generalizing the cognitive, emotional, and overt behavioral and verbal repertoires necessary for effective application of treatment—including the strengthening of therapeutic responses and the reduction of responses that inhibit and/or interfere with effective application of treatment	Supervision, therapist consultation meeting, continuing education, treatment manuals, adherence and competency monitoring, and staff incentives
Structuring the environment through contingency management within the treatment program as a whole as well as through contingency management within the client's community	Clinic director or via administrative interactions, case management, and family and couples interventions

to play needed roles on the team. All team members are asked to share DBT's basic philosophy. Therapy tasks are clearly delegated to different members of the treatment team with the individual therapist and client responsible for seeing that all treatment targets are adequately addressed by someone in the system.

The Role of Skills Training

Individual therapy sessions are typically crowded with high-priority tasks and crises making it difficult to sustain a step-by-step skills training focus. Consequently, skills training is taught in a group format as a class. Linehan (1993b) has taken various evidence-based protocols and distilled them into four categories of skills that clients can learn and practice:

mindfulness, emotion regulation, distress tolerance, and interpersonal effectiveness. Table 1.3 offers a complete list of skills by category. The dialectic of acceptance and change discussed earlier runs through the skills taught to clients. Mindfulness and distress tolerance skills are acceptance oriented. By practicing mindfulness skills, clients become increasingly able to willingly and nonjudgmentally engage with their immediate experience. Mindfulness skills also help clients refrain from impulsive action and when they do act, to act from "wise mind," the intuitive blend of emotion and reason that radically accepts and responds to the moment just as it is. The distress tolerance skills include crisis survival skills which are stopgap measures used to tolerate distress without impulsively doing things that make the situation worse. They also include reality acceptance skills that are psychological and behavioral versions of meditation practices intended to develop a lifestyle of participating with awareness and wisdom.

Emotion regulation and interpersonal effectiveness, on the other hand, are change-oriented skills. Clients learn the natural and adaptive functions of the major emotions and learn practical techniques for preventing emotion dysregulation, for changing or reducing negative emotions, and for increasing positive emotions. They learn how to manage interpersonal conflict, asking for what they want and saying no, in ways that can obtain their objectives while maintaining good relationships and keeping self-respect.

Whenever possible, in session and during coaching calls, the therapist encourages the client to practice replacing dysfunctional responses with appropriate DBT skills. The individual therapist in DBT learns the skills from the inside out, so that from practicing extensively in her own life she can explain how to use the skill in tough circumstances.

The Individual Therapist and the Consultation Team

In comprehensive DBT, each individual therapist participates in a peer-consultation team. The team's role is to help the therapist have the motivation and skills needed to conduct effective therapy. The team helps the therapist clearly conceptualize difficulties in the therapy and remedy these be they the therapist's skills deficits, or his or her own problematic emotions, cognitions, or contingencies that interfere with conducting therapy. This process of peer consultation is a required component of DBT and is described in depth in Chapter 7.

The individual therapist and other members of a DBT consultation team agree to a set of specific assumptions about clients, therapists, and therapy listed in Table 1.4. These are *assumptions*, that is, not statements of fact. They are our agreed-upon default settings for how we'll operate,

TABLE I.3. DBT Skills

Acceptance-oriented skills	Change-oriented skills

Core mindfulness

Taking hold of your mind
- Reasonable mind (logical analysis)
- Emotion mind (emotional experience)
- Wise mind (adding intuitive knowledge to reason and emotion)

"What" skills
- Observe
- Describe
- Participate; allowing experience

"How" skills
- Nonjudgmentally
- One-mindfully
- Effectively

Distress tolerance and acceptance

Crisis survival
- TIP your body chemistry
  - Temperature (ice) of your face
  - Intensely exercise
  - Progressively relax your muscles
- Distract with wise mind: ACCEPTS
  - Activities
  - Contributing
  - Comparisons
  - Emotions (use opposite emotions)
  - Pushing away
  - Thoughts
  - Sensations
- Self-soothe with five senses
  - Taste
  - Smell
  - See
  - Hear
  - Touch
- IMPROVE the moment
  - Imagery
  - Meaning
  - Prayer
  - Relaxation
  - One thing at a time
  - Vacation
  - Encouragement
- Pros and cons
  - Accepting reality
  - Willingness
  - Turning your mind
  - Radical acceptance
  - Mindfulness of current thoughts

Emotion regulation

Changing emotional responses
- Check the facts
- Opposite action (to the emotion)
- Problem solving

Reduce vulnerability: ABC PLEASE
- Accumulate positives
- Build mastery
- Cope ahead of time
- Treat PhysicaL illness
- Balanced Eating
- Avoid mood-altering drugs (unless prescribed by your doctor)
- Balanced Sleep
- Exercise

Interpersonal effectiveness

Objective effectiveness: DEARMAN
- Describe
- Express
- Assert
- Reinforce
- Mindfully
- Appear confident
- Negotiate

Relationship effectiveness: GIVE
- Gentle
- Interested
- Validate
- Easy manner

Self-respect effectiveness: FAST
- Fair
- Avoid apologies
- Stick to values
- Truthful

TABLE 1.4. DBT Assumptions about Clients, Therapy, and Therapists

Assumptions about clients

- Clients are doing the best they can.
- Clients want to improve.
- Clients cannot fail in DBT.
- The lives of suicidal individuals are unbearable as they are currently being lived.
- Clients must learn new behaviors in all relevant contexts.
- Clients may not have caused all of their own problems, but they have to resolve them anyway.
- Clients need to do better, try harder, and/or be more motivated to change.

Assumptions about therapy and therapists

- The most caring thing therapists can do is to help clients change.
- Clarity, precision, and compassion are of the utmost importance in the conduct of DBT.
- The relationship between therapists and clients is a real relationship between equals.
- Therapists can fail to apply the treatment effectively. Even when applied effectively, DBT can fail to achieve the desired outcome.
- Therapists who treat individuals with pervasive emotion dysregulation and Stage 1 behaviors need support.

especially when the chips are down. These assumptions function like a guide rope in a dark twisty cavern, leading the therapist back to empathy for what it is truly like to live in our clients' skins. The assumptions begin with the idea that clients, as with all people, are at any given time doing the best they can and, further, that clients want to improve. Yet, amid setbacks and excruciatingly slow progress it can be easy for us as therapists to communicate frustration, and to act as if the problem is the client's lack of willpower—he or she simply does not want to change badly enough.

But imagine a kid who has practiced indoors all spring to do his first dive off the 10-meter platform. Then on the first beautiful summer day he competes. His family all sit in the audience as he climbs the diving platform. He walks out to the edge, and looks down. A huge wave of fear and vertigo sweep through him. He retreats to the stairs to climb down. He makes eye contact with his dad; the power of his dad's encouraging smile turns him around and moves him back to the edge of the platform. At the edge, he freezes. This is not at all like spring practice: no buddies joking around on the platform with him and no coach talking him through. Just silence as he feels fearful and humiliated. He steps away from the edge. Now, does that kid want to dive? Yes! More than anything. But fear is in the way. The needed behavior has not been practiced in all relevant contexts.

It's like this with our clients. The DBT assumptions, that our clients want to improve and at any given moment are doing the best they can, lead us back to examine factors that interfere with needed behaviors. We assume that new behaviors must be learned in all relevant contexts: what is possible in session in the context of a supportive therapy relationship is different from that which is possible when alone in the middle of the night. Few of us would change places with our most distressed clients—their lives are truly unbearable without change. Yet while clients want to improve and are doing the best they can, often that is not sufficient. He or she in fact must try harder and be more motivated. In essence the boy on the diving board is exactly where he should be: all factors required to create the current circumstance, to have him freeze, trapped between diving or retreating down the stairs, have occurred. Something, somewhere along the way, must go differently for him to dive.

And so we assume it is with our clients: therapy must identify what needs to change in order to have needed behavior occur. The assumption is that even though the client may not have caused all of his or her own problems, he or she must solve them anyway. Here the therapist assumes that the client can't fail but instead views it as the therapist's job and the job of therapy to motivate and enable change. The analogy here is much like chemotherapy: when the patient dies, we don't blame the patient. Rather the assumption is that "treatment fails" because the practitioner failed to follow the protocol or it could be that the treatment itself is inadequate and must be improved. By explicitly agreeing to these assumptions and returning to them the therapist and team avoid unproductive polarization and more rapidly resume a useful stance of phenomenological empathy.

A dialectical stance informs conversations between the therapist and consultation team. This means that polarization is an expected phenomenon, something to be explored rather than avoided. At each point in time, the assumption is that any understanding is partial and likely to leave out something important. For example, a therapist asks for consultation on his work with a client. The team immediately remembers her—she's the one who habitually expresses distress with her husband and her health in an overly dramatic, helpless style that has burnt out all her supportive people. The therapist hasn't talked about this client in weeks. What the team hadn't realized is that, for the last 6 weeks, the client has only sporadically attended individual therapy sessions. The therapist is seeking help now because the client left a message that morning casually informing the therapist that she attempted suicide. The client took a minor overdose of Advil, went to the emergency department, and somehow finagled placement to the city's most plush, supportive day treatment program. The individual therapist flips out in exasperation. While his teammates commiserate and help plan the therapist's next move, somebody on a dialectically informed team will wonder aloud: Has the individual therapist inadvertently shaped the client to communicate distress in this dysfunctional manner because he was not responding to lower-level communications? Has he too burnt out as others have? Someone else on the team will wonder if perhaps the *team* has played a role by shaping the *therapist:* Did the team's impatience with slow progress make the therapist hesitate to ask for help with the client's sporadic attendance and his own sense of burnout? On a dialectically informed team, such dialogues are valued, not viewed as splitting and part of the client's pathology.

The role of the individual therapist—the focus of this book—is to provide psychotherapy and work with the client to make progress toward all treatment goals. While others have input, the individual therapist does the lion's share of treatment planning and crisis management. Next, I outline the framework of treatment priorities that structures the conduct of individual therapy. In DBT, the individual therapist structures therapy based on the extent of client disorder. With highly disordered clients, the therapy environment is highly structured.

Hierarchy of Treatment Goals and Targets for Individual Therapy

The key tool that individual therapists use to structure and prioritize their many therapy tasks is the stage-based hierarchy of treatment goals and targets. *Treatment goals* are the overarching desired end point for a stage of work. *Targets* in DBT are behaviors identified as needing change, whether to be increased or decreased. DBT stages treatment using a commonsense notion: Prioritize problems according to the threat they pose to a reasonable quality of life. Therapy tasks are organized hierarchically so that the most important tasks take priority over the less important. Linehan (1996) has described DBT as a treatment with five stages. Table 1.5 shows the hierarchy of primary targets for pretreatment, Stage 1, and Stage 2 in individual therapy. In addition, there are secondary treatment targets. These address the behavior patterns, the dialectical dilemmas, described earlier. Little has been written and less researched about Stage 3 and Stage 4 of DBT. Linehan says that in Stage 3, the therapist helps the client synthesize what was learned in earlier stages, increase his or her self-respect and the sense of abiding connection, and work toward resolving problems in living. In Stage 4, the therapist focuses on the sense of incompleteness that many individuals experience, even after problems in living are essentially resolved. The task is to give up "ego" and participate fully in the moment with the goal of becoming free of the need for reality to be different from it is at the moment. Although the stages of therapy are presented linearly, progress is often not linear and the stages overlap. When problems arise it is not uncommon to return to discussions like those of pretreatment to regain commitment to the treatment goals or methods. At termination or

TABLE I.5. Hierarchy of Primary and Secondary Targets, by Stage of Individual Psychotherapy

Primary behavioral targets

Pretreatment: Agreement and commitment
• Agreement on goals and methods
• Commitment to complete agreed-upon plan

Stage 1: Severe behavioral dyscontrol → behavioral control

1. Decrease life-threatening behaviors
   • Suicidal or homicidal crisis behaviors
   • Nonsuicidal self-injurious behaviors
   • Suicidal ideation and communications
   • Suicide-related expectancies and beliefs
   • Suicide-related affect
2. Decrease therapy-interfering behaviors
3. Decrease quality-of-life-interfering behaviors
4. Increase behavioral skills
   • Core mindfulness
   • Distress tolerance
   • Interpersonal effectiveness
   • Emotion regulation
   • Self-management

Stage 2: Quiet desperation → emotional experiencing

No a priori hierarchy; instead, prioritized based on individual case formulation

Decrease:
• Intrusive symptoms (e.g., PTSD intrusive symptoms)
• Avoidance of emotions (and behaviors that function as avoidance)
• Avoidance of situations and experiences (i.e., avoidance that includes what is seen in PTSD but that is not specifically limited to avoidance of trauma-related cues)
• Emotion dysregulation (both heightened and inhibited emotional experiencing, specifically related to anxiety/fear, anger, sadness, or shame/guilt)
• Self-invalidation

Secondary behavioral targets (relevant across all stages)

Increase emotion modulation
Decrease emotional reactivity

Increase self-validation
Decrease self-invalidation

Increase realistic decision making and judgment
Decrease crisis-generating behaviors

Increase emotional experiencing
Decrease inhibited grieving

Increase active problem solving
Decrease active passivity

Increase accurate communication of emotions and competencies
Decrease mood dependency of behavior

before breaks, especially if not well prepared, the client may resume Stage 1 behaviors. The transition from Stage 1 to 2 is also difficult for many, because exposure work can lead to intense painful emotions and consequent behavioral dyscontrol. Only pretreatment, Stage 1, and Stage 2 have been well articulated to date and therefore I only cover these three stages in this book.

Pretreatment Stage: Orientation and Commitment

All DBT clients begin in pretreatment. The individual therapist and client use this structured pretreatment phase to formulate the problems the client experiences and tailor a treatment plan. The goals are to learn enough about each other to determine whether they can work together well as a team, agree to the essential goals and methods of treatment, and then to mutually commit to complete the agreed-upon plan of therapy.

Because DBT requires voluntary rather than coerced consent, both the client and the therapist must have the choice of committing to DBT over another non-DBT option. For example, in a forensic unit or when a client is legally mandated to treatment, he or she is not considered to have entered DBT until a considered verbal commitment is obtained. While it is not important to have a written contract, it is important to have a mutual verbal commitment to treatment agreements. Specific agreements may vary by setting and the client's problems. For example, the client might agree to work on identified treatment targets for a specified length of time and to attend all scheduled sessions, pay fees and the like. The therapist might agree to provide the best treatment possible (including increasing their own skills as needed), to abide by ethical principles, and to participate in consultation. In the same manner, therapists on the consultation team undergo a pretreatment process as they consider and agree to consultation team agreements prior to joining the consultation team (described in Chapter 7). All such agreements are in place before beginning formal treatment.

As in any CBT package, orienting strategies (change-oriented) are used to vividly link treatment methods to the client's ultimate goals so that the client understands what is proposed, why it is proposed, and how to do it. Orienting is particularly emphasized in DBT, not only at the beginning of treatment but throughout, because emotion dysregulation may disrupt collaboration with therapy tasks. Even well-considered, gently offered therapist interventions can be experienced as highly invalidating. Consequently, you must frequently explain why a particular treatment task is necessary to reach the client's goals and further, you will need to instruct the client specifically how to do the therapy task despite or in the face of emotion dysregulation. Additionally, many clients enter therapy with implicit expectations about how therapy will proceed based on past therapy experiences. Explicit orientation and socialization about client and therapist roles, responsibilities and expectations can head off misunderstandings and disappointment allowing for well-informed consent before beginning therapy.

Clients often enter the pretreatment stage understandably ambivalent and suspicious about what help therapy can offer given their past treatment failures. Therefore, the client and therapist need to thoroughly discuss concerns and reservations to reach a therapeutic agreement that genuinely works for both parties. The therapist views it as his job to actively assess and enhance the client's motivation starting in pretreatment and throughout therapy whenever needed—this is one of the most important targets of DBT. A number of specific commitment strategies are used in DBT. These are listed in Table 1.1 with other change-oriented strategies. A client is ready to begin Stage 1 if he or she is at least minimally committed to treatment—DBT therapists typically get what they can take, and take what they can get. They work toward gradually shaping greater commitment and motivation throughout the treatment process as I illustrate repeatedly throughout the book.

Stage 1: Attaining Basic Capacities (Reducing Behavioral Dyscontrol)

Stage 1 clients are those with the most severe level of disorder, whose problems and dyscontrol of behavior are so pervasive that they significantly impair quality of life, interfere with therapy, and pose a threat to life. These are the clients that require comprehensive DBT. The primary treatment goals for Stage 1 are to help the client attain the basic capacities he or she needs to stay alive and engaged in treatment, followed by those needed to improve the client's quality of life. The individual therapist allocates treatment time in sessions according to the following priorities: (1) life-threatening behaviors; (2) therapy-interfering behaviors of the therapist or client; (3) behaviors that seriously compromise the client's quality of life; and (4) deficits in behavioral capabilities needed to make life changes.

Within the highest priority category, life-threatening behaviors, priority is further assigned (in descending order of priority) to: suicide or homicide crisis behaviors; nonsuicidal self-injurious behavior; suicidal ideation and communications; suicide-related expectancies and beliefs; and suicide-related affect. These are also listed in Table 1.5. Therapy-interfering behavior is any behavior of either the client or the therapist that negatively affects the therapeutic relationship or that compromises the effectiveness of treatment. For clients this may include missing sessions, excessive psychiatric hospitalization, inability or refusal to work in therapy, and excessive demands on the therapist. For therapists this may include forgetting appointments or being late to them, failing to return phone calls, being inattentive, arbitrarily changing policies, and feeling unmotivated or demoralized about therapy. Quality-of-life targets include any serious mental health problems such as mood or anxiety disorders, substance abuse or eating disorders, psychotic and dissociative phenomena, as well as life problems such as an inability to maintain stable housing, inattention to medical problems, domestic violence, and so on.

The Diary Card

The individual therapist monitors these and other key behaviors through the client's daily completion of a diary card. Review of the card at the start of every session helps the therapist determine what targets may need attention in that session. If the client fails to fill out the card or bring it to the session, it is treated as therapy-interfering behavior. The therapist then works on targets in order of priority by weaving together the core treatment strategies (change, validation, and dialectics). The priority of a target need not always equate with the amount of session time spent on it. The therapist's aim is to get the most progress in each clinical interaction, balancing what is most important with the client's capability and the time available. This is described in detail in Chapter 6.

Priorities for Phone Consultation

The individual therapist is also the main person responsible for seeing that new behaviors are generalized to all relevant environments. The therapist not only uses the therapeutic relationship as a key place for clients to learn and apply new responses but also deliberately structures therapy to ensure what is learned generalizes to all needed contexts. To do this, the therapist uses phone consultation and *in vivo* therapy (i.e., therapy outside the office), which in standard DBT with highly suicidal and emotionally dysregulated clients, is considered essential. There are different priorities for phone calls than for individual therapy sessions. In phone calls, the therapist priorities are (1) decreasing suicide crises behaviors, (2) increasing generalization of skills, and (3) decreasing the sense of conflict, alienation, and distance from the therapist. These coaching calls are brief, typically 5–10 minutes in duration. In addition to phone coaching, the therapist might use milieu skills coaching and treatments, therapeutic communities, *in vivo* interventions (case management), review of session tapes, and systems interventions. This function of generalization can also include family and others in the client's social network (Miller, Rathus,

DuBose, Dexter-Mazza, & Goldberg, 2007; Fruzzetti, Santisteban, & Hoffman, 2007; Porr, 2010). The therapist does what is needed to help the client transfer what is learned in therapy to the client's daily life.

Stage 2: Nontraumatizing Emotional Experience (Decreasing Behaviors Related to Posttraumatic Stress)

As clients stabilize, gain behavioral control, and become more functional, they may enter Stage 2 of treatment (Wagner & Linehan, 2006). In Stage 2, the client works on posttraumatic stress disorder (PTSD) responses and traumatizing emotional experiences. Here the targets may include decreasing intrusive symptoms (e.g., PTSD-intrusive symptoms); avoidance of emotions (and behaviors that function as avoidance) and avoidance of situations and experiences (i.e., avoidance that includes what is seen in PTSD, but that is not specifically limited to avoidance of trauma-related cues); emotion dysregulation (both heightened and inhibited emotional experiencing, specifically related to anxiety/fear, anger, sadness, shame/guilt); and self-invalidation. In contrast to Stage 1 targets, Stage 2 targets are not thought of hierarchically but instead the prioritization of targets is determined by the level of severity and life disruption caused by the problems, the clients' goals, and the functional relationship between targets. For example, if intrusive images provoked an increase in suicidal ideation, they might be prioritized. If, instead, intense self-invalidation and self-loathing were most related to increases in suicidal ideation, that would be prioritized.

Because of the lifetime prevalence of PTSD among treatment-seeking individuals with BPD (36–58%; Linehan, Comtois, Murray, et al., 2006; Zanarini et al., 1998; Zanarini, Frankenburg, Hennen, & Silk, 2004; Zimmerman & Mattia, 1999) and the high incidence of reported new experiences of adult abuse (Zanarini, Frankenburg, Reich, Hennen, & Silk, 2005; Golier et al., 2003), exposure-based CBT protocols such as prolonged exposure should be considered (e.g., Foa et al., 2005; Foa, Rothbaum, Riggs, & Murdock, 1991). However, behaviors common to people with emotion dysregulation are associated unfortunately with poorer outcome in prolonged exposure (e.g., avoidance, severe depression, overwhelming anxiety, guilt, shame, anger, excessive physical tension, numbing, and dissociation; Foa & Kozak, 1986; Foa, Riggs, Massie, & Yarczower, 1995; Jaycox & Foa, 1996; Meadows & Foa, 1998; Feeny, Zoellner, & Foa, 2002; Hembree, Cahill, & Foa, 2004; McDonagh et al., 2005; Zayfert et al., 2005).

Because of their difficulty regulating and tolerating intense emotions, some clients may be at increased risk of impulsive and self-destructive behaviors during exposure-based therapy. Therefore, in DBT, the client and therapist are encouraged to carefully assess readiness to engage in exposure-based therapy (Stage 2). Tentatively, indicators of readiness include: the ability to control suicidal and nonsuicidal self-injurious behavior (e.g., abstinence from these behaviors for 2–4 months); a firm commitment not to engage in these behaviors in the future; and demonstrated ability to use skills to effectively manage urges to engage in these behaviors. The client and therapist might test whether the client is ready to begin Stage 2 work by choosing an item from the exposure hierarchy that is of low distress and see how he or she manages it. Exposure may be contraindicated when the client cannot be exposed to the trauma cues without dissociating or is currently experiencing crises or logistical issues that would block participation in treatment.

Many treatment development efforts are under way to adapt exposure-based procedures for individuals with pervasive emotion dysregulation and suicidal behaviors, including techniques designed to improve distress tolerance, further titrate anxiety and other emotions during exposure, and manage suicidality. For those with less severe disorder (e.g., those without suicidal and nonsuicidal self-injurious behavior) an abbreviated course of DBT skills training prior to exposure (e.g., Cloitre et al., 2002), a DBT-informed exposure treatment (e.g., Becker & Zayfert, 2001; Zayfert et al., 2005), or a standard exposure treatment without any priming intervention might work. Harned and Linehan's (2008) preliminary data suggest that clients quite early in Stage 1 DBT can in fact successfully participate in prolonged exposure for PTSD if they are well oriented, behavior is stabilized, and sufficient emotion regulation skills have been acquired. It's to be expected that clients may continue to experience low to moderate urges to self-injure or attempt suicide while undergoing exposure treatment. If these urges become too intense, exposure therapy may need to be temporarily postponed while the primary therapist helps the client regain or strengthen behavioral control. For this reason it may be helpful to have a different therapist conduct exposure therapy while the individual therapist continues his or her usual DBT sessions in tandem with the exposure work.

By staging treatment based on the extent of the client's disorder and prioritizing client behavioral problems, the therapist stays clear on the highest priorities, even in chaotic circumstances. Across all stages, DBT emphasizes learning to regulate emotion. While the amount of structure in the treatment environment depends on the extent of client disorder, the biosocial theory and core strategies remain steady. Applying the core strategies of DBT—change, validation, and dialectics—may initially appear straightforward, but the devil is in the details. In ever-changing, often high-risk and emotionally challenging clinical situations, applying even straightforward concepts becomes complicated. The nearly infinite if–then circumstances of clinical work mean that you often are working from several sets of principles simultaneously. Any given moment is like hand-weaving an intricate tapestry. It's daunting, holding all the threads, working the tiny section that's immediately before you yet moving with the overall picture in mind. In fact, when Linehan first began to teach DBT, others who saw her clinical demonstrations often said to her, "you're a gifted therapist. You have an amazingly effective personal style and understanding of these patients, but no one else could pull that off." And yet hundreds of therapists, with training and practice, have indeed "pulled it off." As Malcolm Gladwell (2008) argues in his analysis of outstanding performers, while some innate talent is important, it's not talent that explains performance differences and good outcomes. It's practice. And the first thing to practice is how to conceptualize the client's problems using the principles of DBT. In Chapter 2, I'll describe how case formulation is used in DBT to structure the therapist's clinical decision making and treatment planning for an individual client. Whether you use the full comprehensive model of DBT or instead use its philosophy and strategies to inform your therapy, case formulation is the individual therapist's first step.

TWO

Navigating to a Case Formulation and Treatment Plan

This chapter describes how DBT uses theory-driven case formulation for treatment planning and clinical decision making. A case formulation is a set of hypotheses about the causes of a person's difficulties; it helps you to translate general treatment protocols into an individualized treatment plan. Terms like "formulation" and "treatment plan" tend to imply static documents, like maps. However, DBT case conceptualization and treatment planning must be *active*.

Good basic treatment models, like good maps, can help you navigate a lot of terrain. For example, you can use Barlow's unified protocol (Allen, McHugh, & Barlow, 2008) to generate a formulation and treatment plan whether the client fears and avoids spiders, social rejection, or his own disturbing thoughts or bodily sensations. You still may need to tailor assessment and exposure exercises for a particular client. But navigating to a conceptualization and treatment plan in these circumstances is like finding an on ramp on a sunny day—with your map and a friendly point in the right direction, you're on your way in no time.

Finding your way becomes exponentially more complicated when a person has multiple, chronic serious problems. You're often in uncharted territory where neither the research literature nor local colleagues can offer confident direction. Further, the usual ways you evaluate whether therapy is on the right track don't work because your interventions are experienced as intensely invalidating and evoke extreme emotional dysregulation. Making sense of what is going on and what is needed is much like traveling in a blizzard with whiteout conditions; you may sense forward motion, but often cannot get your bearings to be sure that it is meaningful progress.

Therefore in DBT, you must be active. Orienteering is the best metaphor for formulating DBT cases and planning treatment, because it conveys the level of activity required to find your way from point *A* to point *B*. You need to be able to read your client, to locate where you are, and to use relevant science and treatments that offer direction. You also must continually check your bearings, revise your route if needed, yet stay focused on the destination. The number and complexity of obstacles encountered en route require increasingly flexible yet disciplined navigation. Three sets of concepts, introduced in Chapter 1, help us navigate in DBT:

- Target hierarchies prioritize what to assess and treat based on the severity of clients' problems.
- Biosocial theory is used to understand the core problem of pervasive emotion dysregulation. We assume that (1) biological vulnerability and social invalidation are contributing factors to emotion dysregulation; and (2) primary and secondary target behaviors are likely consequences of emotion dysregulation (e.g., dissociation) or they function as the client's solutions to the problem of emotion dysregulation (i.e., provide temporary relief from aversive states).
- Behavioral theories of change are used to identify the controlling variables and contributing factors for primary target behaviors. These include invalidation and emotion dysregulation, specific skills deficits, problematic conditioned emotional responses, contingencies, or cognitive factors. Behavioral theories guide interventions used to strengthen more adaptive alternative responses.

We use these concepts dialectically to formulate problems and plan treatment. The key idea here is: truth evolves. The individual therapist does not find his or her way by reasoning from an immutable set of facts. But neither is clinical reasoning a relativistic process where anything goes. Instead, you take a dialectical stance. This means that you enter a series of dialogues, with the client and others important to your work together, such as the client's significant others and the consultation team. These conversations are informed by the scientific evidence base and the life experiences of each of you. These dialogues lead to syntheses. As you formulate the client's problems, you can only hold a part of the "truth." Perspectives of others (e.g., the client's parent or psychiatrist) or direct observations of the client at different points in time (e.g., in a good mood vs. in a crisis state) are all parts of a greater whole. What is known from science about "the average client" may or may not apply to this specific person; what is "known" changes over time. Any understanding is likely partial and likely to leave something important out yet through dialogues we experience the contradictions inherent in our own position—through dialogues we reach more whole and coherent truths that help us change.

In other words, the purpose of case formulation and treatment planning in DBT is not to reach some ultimate "correct" understanding but instead to constructively face the tension of opposing formulations; rather than choose one at the expense of the other, the tension is used to create a third more complete model from what is valid in each position. For example, say a client struggles with social phobia. Catching a bus to participate in skills training group is very difficult (although she does get to church via bus some Sundays). Should the treatment plan be based on accepting her vulnerability and therefore remove the requirement of group attendance or should it block avoidance by insisting on attendance to help her make needed change? In formulating this dilemma in DBT, you would take the position that attending group is overwhelmingly difficult *and* attending group is required. Dialectical assessment and treatment planning would hold both positions simultaneously so that solutions incorporate what is valid from each. For example, the initial treatment plan might be based on accepting that the client's current capabilities preclude regularly riding the bus to group and simultaneously move for change by offering *in vivo* skills coaching each week on the bus to group. Similarly, change is at times so slow and the client's distress so unremitting that you can't be sure if you are persisting with an ineffective treatment plan or whether in fact the therapy is going as well as it could given the circumstances and you should stay the course. In DBT the idea is that rather than prematurely taking one position (therapy isn't working; therapy is working) you instead hold both positions in mind at once, searching for what is valid in each with the stance that truth evolves. Seemingly contradictory elements can be synthesized and something is bound to be left out of any current understanding.

Practically, formulating and planning treatment works best if you use the above concepts in three steps. First, you assess to determine the appropriate stage of treatment based on the extent to which the client's behavior is disordered. In particular look for instances of pretreatment and Stage 1 target behaviors. Second, look for the variables that control these pretreatment and Stage 1 primary targets. In particular, biosocial theory points us toward invalidation or other events that may set off emotion dysregulation. Look especially for patterns across targets and over time. Finally use solution analysis and task analysis to generate mini-treatment plans for changing the key variables that drive primary targets.

Let's now go step by step to show how to generate an initial formulation, and then how to use the formulation to guide clinical interactions.

STEP 1: ASSESS USING STAGES
AND TREATMENT TARGETS

Your first step toward a formulation and treatment plan is to gather sufficient history to determine the appropriate stage of treatment. This crucial step determines whether comprehensive treatment will be needed to adequately help the client. Even upon first contact, let your standard intake assessment questions be guided by the framework of stages and primary targets described in Chapter 1. Stage treatment to match the extent to which the client's behavior is disordered. Table 2.1 shows examples of potential intake questions organized according to target hierarchy. When you ask, for example, "What has brought you to therapy now?" you listen with the target hierarchy in the back of your mind. At an appropriate moment, you might ask explicitly for information about each target area—for example, "Have things gotten so bad you've been thinking a lot about death or even about killing yourself?" "How have things gone for you in past therapy?"

If the client's responses seem to fit one of the stages of treatment (e.g., Stage 1, "yes, I tried to kill myself and ended up in intensive care" or "things blew up with my last therapist," or "I've had a lot of therapy and nothing seems to change, I don't have much hope for therapy but don't know what else to do"), then use the corresponding target hierarchy to guide further assessment of each target area. For example, if the person sounds ambivalent about changing a particular behavior or about therapy itself, use pretreatment targets to guide questions. If the person has thought a lot about death, thought she would be better off dead, or has had mixed results in past attempts at therapy, then begin to use Stage 1 targets to generate questions about a more comprehensive list of problems. What difficulties (if any) have clients had with intentional self-injury and other life-threatening behavior? How have past therapies gone and what's gotten in the way of getting the help they've needed from therapists and others in their lives? When clients have had histories of failed therapies, be sure to assess what functions of comprehensive treatment might have been missing or problematic (e.g., was there enough attention to increasing skills and generalization, sufficient one-to-one work on motivation, did the therapist receive adequate support?). What significant quality-of-life problems does the person struggle with? Assess each. Finally, what skills does the person need but lack? DBT skills training is geared toward common deficits in mindfulness, emotion regulation, distress tolerance, and interpersonal effectiveness. Listen for evidence that skills deficits in one or more of these areas play an important role in the client's problems.

TABLE 2.1. Assessment Questions and Resources by Stage and Target

Pretreatment

Can the therapist and client agree to:
• Goals of treatment?
• Methods of treatment?

Can the therapist and client commit to fulfill all agreements?
What barriers (if any) are there to:
• Agreement on the therapy goals and methods?
• Sufficient commitment to treatment?

Define any disagreement or ambivalence on the part of either party. Assess controlling variables. Work toward agreement and commitment.

Stage 1

Is there any risk of life-threatening behavior?

Intentional self-injury?

(To client:) Have things gotten so bad that you've thought a lot about death or that you believe you'd be better off dead?

(To client:) Have you ever tried to kill yourself? Have you ever intentionally injured yourself?

Scan for suicide crises, nonsuicidal self-injurious behavior, suicidal ideation, suicide-related expectancies and beliefs, suicide-related affect. Especially assess near lethal suicide attempts, acts of self-injury with high intent to die, and other medically serious self-injurious behavior.

What behaviors of the client and the therapist may interfere with therapy?

If past treatment was a failure, was it attributable in part to a lack of comprehensive treatment (i.e., were all five functions provided)?

(To client:) How have things gone for you in past therapy? What has gotten in the way of getting the help you needed?

(Therapist/treatment team:) Assess whether all five functions were delivered in past therapies.

What serious chronic problems interfere with the client's quality of life?

What skills deficits hinder the client?

Stage 2

Is emotional experience itself traumatizing?

Are there PTSD responses that interfere with the client's quality of life?

Now consider two individuals, Samantha and Jonelle, who are new referrals to a DBT practice. Let's walk through how to assess the appropriate stage of treatment during an intake or initial session.

Samantha

Background and History

Samantha is a 24-year-old who was referred to the DBT program from the state psychiatric hospital. She cuts and burns her arms and legs, and has overdosed on pain killers with ambivalent intent to die ("if it happens, it happens; it's like Russian roulette"). She takes opiates for chronic back pain; at 21 she was hit head on by a drunk driver, and suffered severe injuries. Her passenger died in the accident. She has struggled with bulimia and cutting since she was 16, but after the accident, her intent to die and suicidal behavior became worse and the disordered eating more medically serious. She binges and purges and most recently purged to the extent that she induced heart problems that prompted admission to her nearby rural medical hospital. When medically stabilized, she transferred to the state hospital. The therapist hears from the person referring her that Samantha and the state hospital staff moved mountains to arrange for Samantha to live with an aunt in order to be able to work with the DBT program.

Thinking in terms of stage of treatment helps the therapist to organize what she knows so far. How might the therapist answer the questions in Table 2.1 given just Samantha's background and history? Here is her preliminary thinking.

Pretreatment: Can Client and Therapist Reach Agreement on Therapy Goals and Methods? What Barriers (If Any) Are There to Sufficient Commitment to Treatment?

The effort by the client, her family, and the state hospital staff to arrange the first appointment indicates some degree of commitment already. The highest pretreatment stage priority for initial sessions will be to assess Samantha's goals, including: her desire to stop suicidal behavior and other intentional self-injury, to stop disordered eating, and her willingness to learn alternative methods to manage intense emotions.

Stage I: Is There Risk from Life-Threatening Behavior?

Thorough assessment is definitely needed here. A DBT therapist wants details about five types of life-threatening behavior (in descending order of priority): (1) suicide crisis behaviors; (2) nonsuicidal self-injurious behavior; (3) suicidal ideation and communications; (4) suicide-related expectancies and beliefs; and (5) suicide-related affect. Either before treatment or early in treatment, the therapist needs to gather details regarding intentional self-injury for the past year, including exactly what was done, the intent of the action, and whether medical attention was required. This history is essential to assess suicide risk accurately, to begin to identify situations that evoke suicide ideation and intentional self-injury, and to manage suicidal crises. In particular, the therapist needs to identify the conditions associated with (1) near-lethal suicide attempts, (2) other acts of self-injury with high intent to die, and (3) other medically serious self-injurious behavior. The information we have about Samantha definitely indicates that further assessment here is needed.

Stage 1: Is There Any History of Therapy-Interfering Behavior?

This second primary target of Stage 1, treatment-interfering behaviors, includes behavior of either the client or the therapist that negatively affects the therapeutic relationship or that compromises the effectiveness of treatment, as described in Chapter 1. Information about these targets should be obtained from prior treatment history and prior supervision history. We don't have much information yet about Samantha's treatment history so we will want to gather that. The consultation team helps the therapist anticipate his or her own therapy-interfering behavior in a new therapy relationship. If Samantha were a new client in your practice, what therapy-interfering behavior might you be likely to bring to the therapy? What are your usual foibles (e.g., running late, having too narrow limits), and what might be specifically evoked by Samantha's problems (e.g., not being up to date on assessment and treatment of PTSD or pain; biases you have because you are a parent of children about Samantha's age)?

Stage 1: Are There Behaviors That Seriously Impair the Client's Quality of Life?

The quickest way to assess the third primary target area, quality of life, would be a diagnostic evaluation and thorough psychosocial history to understand the range of problems Samantha experiences. Assess how problems like mood and anxiety disorders, substance abuse, eating disorders, psychotic and dissociative phenomena, an inability to maintain stable housing, and inattention to medical problems, and so on, may impair a client's quality of life, influence intentional self-injury, and also interfere with therapy. So far, the therapist knows that she wants to assess

Samantha's disordered eating, chronic pain and use of narcotics, her use of the hospital, and the stability of her living situation.

Because Samantha survived a car accident when others did not and because her problems worsened after the accident, the therapist will want to assess for PTSD. Treatment of PTSD is typically deferred until Stage 2, when a client has sufficient emotion regulation and behavioral control to manage the increased emotion evoked. However, in Samantha's case we want to determine whether there is a functional relationship between the accident and her current difficulties. Might some of her current Stage 1 behaviors function to avoid or regulate emotions or memories to do with the accident? If remembering the accident continues to affect her and is linked to intentional self-injury, these factors might become Stage 1 priority targets. However, if exposure-based procedures were indicated, assessment and caution are needed to ensure that the client does not use Stage 1 behaviors to cope with the increased experience of emotion (Harned & Linehan, 2008). If Samantha's behavior became more unstable or urges to intentionally self-injure became more difficult to control when the therapist talked about the accident, it would indicate that Stage 1 targets should be addressed before those of Stage 2. The infrequency of Stage 1 behaviors as well as the speed of re-regulation (rather than the presence of any one instance of behavior) would determine whether Samantha is ready for directly targeting PTSD responses. Samantha and her therapist should likely test the waters by talking about some aspect of the trauma that is of low distress to see if Samantha can safely tolerate exposure.

Jonelle

Background and History

Now consider Jonelle, who found the therapist's name on the Internet. She is a 28-year-old legal secretary. When first speaking with her on the phone, the therapist learns that her 4-year-old son has been kicked out of his second day care center due to conduct and attention problems. She and her son are living with Jonelle's mother, who endlessly criticizes Jonelle's parenting. Jonelle says she feels paranoid and humiliated by her mother talking with all the neighbors about her "crazy" daughter. Arguments with her mother and her mother's boyfriend have gotten so loud that neighbors have called the police. In the last argument, Jonelle became intensely angry, locked herself in the bathroom, and punched her legs until she calmed down. At that time, Jonelle said she seriously considered suicide and even poured her mother's heart medication and sleeping pills into her hand. But the realization of how it would impact her son made her stop. She said the one good thing that came out of that dark moment was the clarity that suicide would never again be an option for her.

When the therapist offers her a late afternoon appointment, Jonelle balks because she is concerned about taking time off from a new demanding job; the cost of therapy is also hard because she is paying back student loans. The therapist's policy of charging for sessions cancelled without 24-hour notice also doesn't work for her, given how frequently she has to deal with her son's misbehavior. She saw on the Internet that DBT has a group therapy component, and the idea of going to group therapy turns her off. When the therapist acknowledges how difficult things are for her, she says: "Yes, what I really need is to get married. That would get me out of this house, money to pay my loans, and somebody who could control my son."

Let's see how the therapist uses the target hierarchy to organize what she knows of Jonelle's struggles.

Pretreatment: Can Client and Therapist Reach Agreement on Therapy Goals and Methods? What Barriers (If Any) Are There to Sufficient Commitment to Treatment?

Jonelle is understandably ambivalent about spending time and money on therapy, given her finances, new-hire status, and responsibilities as a parent. You would definitely want to assess and address the reservations Jonelle has as well as clarify her therapy goals. DBT may be one possible treatment recommendation for Jonelle, based on the data the therapist has so far. That data include her report of one instance of a suicide crisis and intentional self-injury, seemingly precipitated by invalidation and difficulty with emotion regulation, but the therapist doesn't yet know whether this is a pattern for her. Further assessment may show that an equally valid treatment option would be time-limited therapy focused on moving out of her mother's house. It might also be focused on parenting training to help Jonelle and her mother negotiate conflicts about her difficult-to-raise son. Only further assessment will show whether Jonelle fits Stage 1 and therefore needs comprehensive treatment.

Stage 1: Is There Risk from Life-Threatening Behavior?

Assess the categories of nonsuicidal self-injury and suicidal behavior as described above (suicide crisis behaviors; nonsuicidal self-injurious behavior; suicidal ideation and communications; suicide-related expectancies and beliefs; and suicide-related affect). In particular, you would like to understand how determined she feels that she would never attempt suicide again. You would also want to assess the potential for physical aggression toward her mother and perhaps her son. Again, if this was an isolated crisis, you might include elements of DBT in a treatment plan rather than offer the comprehensive model. However, if there are several instances of suicide crises or intentional self-injury, comprehensive DBT may be an option for Jonelle to consider.

Stage 1: Is There Any History of Therapy-Interfering Behavior?

There is great likelihood of therapy-interfering behavior—Jonelle's circumstances already indicate that this will be an important area to discuss with her. As a parent of a young son with behavior problems, she may need the option to cancel at the last minute. As a recent college graduate repaying student loans, she may need a sliding scale fee. She is lukewarm about group skills training, and here again the therapist will need to understand and work out with Jonelle how to solve the barriers if they decide this is a crucial element of the treatment plan. The therapist will need to be clear how her own limits fit Jonelle's needs for flexibility. They need to come to mutually agreeable solutions prior to beginning therapy.

Stage 1: Are There Behaviors That Seriously Impair the Client's Quality of Life?

A good diagnostic interview and psychosocial history will be needed with details about each of the primary target areas. This can determine whether Jonelle's difficulties are the result of a more discrete situational conflict or a pervasive pattern. The mantra is to "Assess, not assume."

As these two case examples show, target hierarchies guide you from the first moments of contact, to determine the focus of treatment and how comprehensive treatment may need to be.

STEP 2: LOOK FOR PATTERNS OF CONTROLLING VARIABLES FOR EACH PRIMARY TARGET

When a particular target area is relevant for a client, select specific instances of that target behavior and use chain analysis to identify the controlling variables; these are the conditions that give rise to and maintain problem behaviors and improvements. Behavioral assessment (cf. Haynes & O'Brien, 2000) puts a premium on identifying controlling variables. The assumption is that each individual's problematic behavior is likely to be controlled by a unique pattern of variables, and these variables may differ from one set of circumstances to another. For example, the factors that lead one individual to attempt suicide are different from those of another individual. Even for the same individual, what led to one attempt might be different from a later attempt. Therefore, to understand a specific disordered or problematic behavior, DBT relies on a particularly fine-grained method of functional analysis called chain analysis.

Behavioral Chain Analysis

A behavioral chain analysis is an in-depth analysis of events and contextual factors before and after an instance (or set of instances) of the targeted behavior. It is a way to identify the controlling variables for the behavior. You and the client together develop a reasonably complete account. The focus is pragmatic: what would be needed for the sequence of events to go differently so that the problem behavior did not occur and instead the client could have a more desired outcome?

Steps in Conducting a Chain Analysis

Begin the chain analysis by clearly defining the *problem behavior* and picking one instance to analyze. For example, a problem behavior might be that a client burst into tears when a supervisor criticized her work yesterday. Next, the therapist and client identify two important types of controlling variables: precipitating events and vulnerability factors. *Precipitating events* are the immediate events that began the chain that led to the problem behavior. *Vulnerability factors* create a context in which precipitating events have more influence, for example, physical illness, sleep deprivation, or other conditions that influence emotional reactivity. In our example, the supervisor's criticism is the precipitating event. Typically, this might be a relative nonevent that sets off mild irritation. However, in the context of two vulnerability factors, being sleep deprived and on a tight deadline, the criticism precipitates bursting into tears. Vulnerability factors set the context for precipitating events to have more power.

Next, the therapist and client identify each *link* between the precipitating event and the problematic behavior to yield a detailed account of each thought, feeling, and action that moved the client from point *A* to point *B*. Close attention is paid to reciprocal interactions between environmental events and the client's emotional, cognitive, and overt responses. Finally, the therapist and client identify the *consequences* associated with the problem behavior—those immediate and delayed reactions of the client and others that followed the problem behavior. It is helpful to visually chart chain analyses. Figure 2.1 illustrates one way to diagram the elements of a chain analysis.

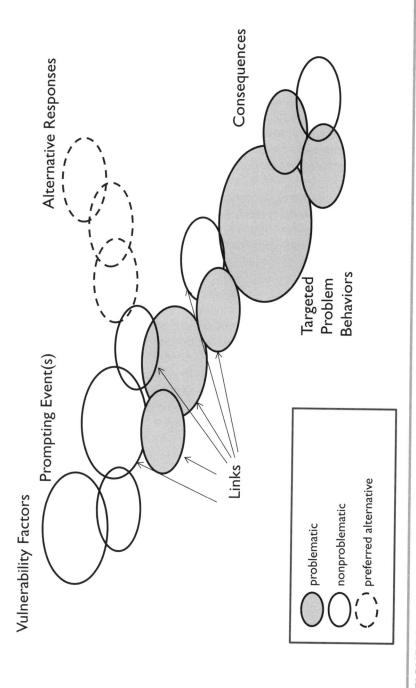

Vulnerability Factors

Prompting Event(s)

Alternative Responses

Consequences

Targeted Problem Behaviors

Links

problematic
nonproblematic
preferred alternative

FIGURE 2.1. Elements of behavioral chain analysis.

Chain Analysis of Jonelle's Suicidal Behavior

Let's look now at the chain analysis for Jonelle's most recent intentional suicide crisis behavior. Figure 2.2 shows how this was diagrammed. In the session with Jonelle, the therapist began with the problem behavior— preparing to overdose on her mother's pills—and then worked with Jonelle to detail what led up to that point and what followed it. Jonelle told the story chronologically as follows.

The precipitating event began mid-morning, when Jonelle's son was home sick from day care, causing her to miss work at her new job. Her son was already complaining of being bored and was rummaging around in Jonelle's bedroom closet. As Jonelle turned to ask him to find something else to do, she felt her mother come and pause at the bedroom door behind her to watch the interaction (precipitating event). Jonelle said this put her on "edge." She said she had been about to say to her son, "Five more minutes, and then you need to play somewhere else," but with her mother at the door she instead said in a tense voice, "Come out, I don't need you playing in my closet." The diagram then shows the further cascade of thoughts, emotions, actions, and events that link the precipitating event to the targeted problem behavior.

As she waited for him to comply, Jonelle said she imagined hearing her mother say, "You have to be firm with him, Jonelle." She had a flood of emotions: irritation and fear as she anticipated her mother's criticism; shame that she "can't get him to mind"; hurt that her mother, of all people, was not more understanding of how hard it was to parent the boy; dread in the pit of her stomach; and a sense of feeling trapped. Her son ignored her request. Without thinking, she harshly yelled, "I said *get out* of there!" Her mother then walked to the closet and said in a gentle voice to the boy, "Come on, honey, let's get you out of your mother's hair." This comment felt extremely critical to Jonelle—her mother's indirect way of saying Jonelle was overreacting and that she needed to protect the son from Jonelle. It felt as if her mother had said to her son, "Your mother's crazy, be quiet and tiptoe around her so you don't set her off."

Jonelle felt furious and viewed her mother as undermining her authority. Jonelle then snapped at her mother, they began arguing, and the son ran from the room crying. Jonelle's mother then said, "Look what you did! You are scaring that boy out of his mind!" Jonelle said at this point she saw red and had an intense urge to grab her mother by the throat and strangle her. Instead, she screamed in frustration and punched her fist through the flimsy bedroom door.

As she felt herself getting more and more out of control, she stumbled past her mother into the bathroom and locked herself in. She sat on the toilet seat and repeatedly pounded her fists into her thighs "to punish"

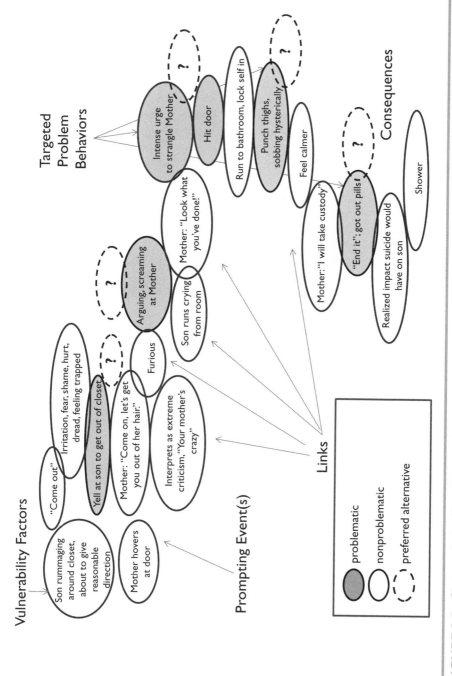

Vulnerability Factors

Prompting Event(s)

Links

Targeted Problem Behaviors

Consequences

Son rummaging around closet, about to give reasonable direction

Mother hovers at door

"Come out"

Irritation, fear, shame, hurt, dread, feeling trapped

Yell at son to get out of closet

Mother: "Come on, let's get you out of her hair."

Interprets as extreme criticism, "Your mother's crazy"

Furious

?

Arguing, screaming at Mother

?

Son runs crying from room

Mother: "Look what you've done!"

Intense urge to strangle Mother

?

Hit door

Run to bathroom, lock self in

Punch thighs, sobbing hysterically

?

Feel calmer

Mother: "I will take custody"

"End it"; got out pills

?

Realized impact suicide would have on son

Shower

problematic

nonproblematic

preferred alternative

FIGURE 2.2. Chain analysis of Jonelle's suicide crisis.

herself and get herself to "calm down." Jonelle said she was sobbing hysterically at the beginning but had calmed down after about 5 minutes of hitting herself. Then her mother came to the bathroom door and said, "I am going to call child protective services and find out how to get custody and take my grandson away from you." When her mother said this, Jonelle suddenly felt very calm. She said she had this sense that she could end it and her mother would look after her son. She said through the door, "I know you love my son. You do what you need to do. I just need some time to think now, OK? Just give me some peace." She emptied her mother's heart medication and sleep medication onto the bathroom counter, got a glass of water, and then turned on the shower so her mother would not interrupt her (targeted problem behavior of planning suicide attempt). She said she got scared and also had thoughts about her son and what her suicide might do to his life. Then with great clarity, she realized she could never do that to him. She took a shower until the water ran cold. Afterward she went to the kitchen and her mother said "either you get help or you get out of here and I am going to take custody of this boy" (consequences).

Looking for Controlling Variables in the Chain Analysis

As mentioned above, a detailed chain analysis allows the therapist to identify each juncture where an alternative client response might have led away from problem behavior. The target hierarchy, biosocial theory, and behavioral theories of change each help guide the process of identifying the controlling variables.

First, the target hierarchy tells us that the priorities are: to assess and treat the factors leading toward suicidal behavior (gathering her mother's medications in preparation for an overdose) and then, next, toward self-injurious behavior (punching her legs) and to understand the potential for violence (toward her mother). Note that each of these important problem behaviors could in its own right be the target of a chain analysis. However, because in this example we are focusing on the highest priority of suicidal behavior, the problem behaviors of punching her leg and the near-violent argument with her mother are viewed as links along the chain that led to suicidal behavior.

Second, biosocial theory tells us to look for emotion dysregulation and invalidation as antecedents to these suicidal and self-injurious behaviors. Invalidation from her mother does seem to have contributed to Jonelle's emotional dysregulation. Biosocial theory also suggests that primary target behaviors may be a result of the overwhelming emotional state or may function to end overwhelming emotional states. Jonelle describes both. At times she feels so out of control that she will lash out at anything (out-of-control behavior is part of extremely dysregulated emotion). At other times, she deliberately hits herself in order to feel calmer (dysfunctional behavior works to regulate emotion).

Third, behavioral theories of change suggest that dysfunctional responses come from one or more of four factors: skills deficits, problematic conditioned emotional reactions, contingencies, or cognitive processes. The blends of these factors are infinite as with sweet, salty, sour, and bitter flavors. Look systematically at the possible role each of these factors may play in leading up to and following target behaviors in the chain analysis.

Skills Deficits

First, assess whether the client has the necessary skills in his or her repertoire. Can the client (1) regulate emotions, (2) tolerate distress, (3) respond skillfully to interpersonal conflict, and (4) observe, describe, and participate without judging, with awareness, and focusing on effectiveness? When clients lack a needed skill, skills training is appropriate. For example, one hypothesis is that Jonelle lacks assertiveness skills—for example, she is not able to ask her mother to stop hovering at the door. The therapist assesses this further across situations and across time. It turns out that Jonelle typically avoids conflict with her mother, acquiescing, feeling resentful—and then eventually blows up. The same pattern holds with past lovers. At work, however, while she avoids conflict, she has always avoided blowups. Across situations, she seldom observes her limits or asks for what she wants—skills deficits may in fact be contributing here. Another hypothesis is that Jonelle lacks skills to soothe physiology, tolerate distress, and downregulate emotion. In the initial interview, Jonelle described being a sensitive child and said that as a teenager she used to get high all the time to be able to tolerate her mother. Now that she's clean and sober, her mother is constantly on her nerves; she feels so irritable and jumpy that she can't stand to be in her own skin. Here, too, skills deficits may be a key variable: if Jonelle had reliable and diverse ways to tolerate and manage emotional arousal, it might offer an important way off the chain and away from the primary target behaviors.

You can assess whether a person has relevant skills in several ways. You might ask the client for details about how a problem or interaction has been handled in the past under varying circumstances. You could observe the client's behavior directly. You can ask hypothetically how the client would ideally handle a situation or problem or what advice they would give a friend. Or you can ask the client to try new behaviors during session and in role-plays. In our example, the therapist assessed Jonelle's parenting skills, by gathering history as well as by directly overhearing

Jonelle parent her son during coaching calls. The therapist learned that Jonelle and her son experienced very little conflict on weekends when Jonelle's mother was away visiting relatives. Jonelle had effective parenting skills even with a very spirited child—the problem seemed to be accessing the skills in the face of anticipated or actual criticism from her mother. The skill she lacked was the ability to regulate her emotion when criticized. Jonelle also could not effectively assert herself with her domineering mother.

When assessment reveals that the client *can* perform skillfully, then the therapist assesses which of the three other factors interfered with using or choosing more skillful behavior.

Conditioned Emotional Responses

Sometimes conditioned emotional responses block more skillful responding. Effective behaviors may be inhibited or disorganized by shame, guilt, unwarranted fears, or other intense or out-of-control emotions. The person may be "emotion-phobic." She or he may have patterns of avoidance or escape behaviors. If this is the case, then some version of exposure-based treatment is indicated. This is a key hypothesis for Jonelle. As the therapist became more detailed in the chain analysis, it turned out that shame was the primary emotion. When her mother was at the door and then again when her mother said to the boy, "let's get you out of your mother's hair," shame flooded Jonelle. Anger was the secondary response. Consequently, principles of exposure therapy will offer an important pathway to change her emotional reactions so they are more regulated, enabling her to access her skillful parenting.

Problematic Contingencies

Skilled performance may be absent because circumstances reinforce dysfunctional behavior or fail to reinforce more functional behavior. Effective behaviors may be followed by neutral or punishing outcomes, or rewarding outcomes may be delayed. For example, Jonelle's effective parenting is often immediately followed by her mother's comment, "See, that wasn't so hard! Why can't you do it that way all the time?" Over time, this aversive consequence has decreased the probability of Jonelle's effective parenting when her mother is around. Problem behavior may lead to positive or preferred outcomes, or give the opportunity for preferred behaviors or emotional states. For example, intentional self-injury often generates desirable consequences (e.g., functions as self-punishment, communicates distress to others, provides pain analgesia through release of endogenous opiates, Nock, 2009). When self-harm functions to communicate distress and then is followed by increased responsiveness of others in the environment, the likelihood of future self-injury may increase. Said differently, nonsuicidal self-injury may be maintained by positive reinforcement. However, intentional self-injury often also is maintained by negative reinforcement. It ends aversive states, such as negative emotions or the tension as one struggles against urges to cut. Jonelle experienced great calm and relief after she punched herself and also when she fantasized about taking an overdose. The same individual may have both types of contingencies controlling intentional self-injury. When Jonelle first began to hit herself as a child, her teachers were solicitous (positive reinforcement) and her mother would stop verbally attacking (negative reinforcement). If problematic contingencies maintain the target behavior, then use contingency management interventions.

Problematic Cognitive Processes or Content

The fourth possibility is that effective behaviors are inhibited by patterns of problematic thinking, or specific faulty beliefs and assumptions. If problems are identified here, then cognitive modification strategies are appropriate. It's tempting to assume that Jonelle is overreacting because she misinterprets or distorts her mother's comment ("she's calling me crazy in front of my son") and to consider cognitive modification to decrease anger (e.g., to find alternative interpretations such as that her mother's intent was helpful, even if unwelcome). Rather than assume, the therapist assessed this further and in fact found that Jonelle's mother is extremely verbally abusive—if anything, Jonelle minimized rather than exaggerated the invalidation. Instead of cognitive restructuring to modify misinterpretations and help Jonelle be less angry, the hypothesis instead here is that Jonelle needs help believing she has the right to appropriately assert her needs even when others are displeased and critical.

Such detailed chain analysis shows the client and therapist junctures where an alternative client response might have led toward the ultimate change the client wants. When the client's responses are dysfunctional (the responses interfere with achieving the client's long-term goals), the therapist assesses what alternative behavior would have been more functional and why that more skillful alternative did not happen. Jonelle and her therapist identified three junctures as most important. In Figure 2.3, dysfunctional response links are phrased in terms of change goals that Jonelle endorsed. They agreed to find replacement behaviors so that (1) no matter how extreme her mother's invalidation, Jonelle will not resort to suicidal behavior or intentional self-injury; (2) Jonelle will be able to handle the conflict with her mother in a way that does not upset her son; and (3) although almost beyond her ability to imagine, Jonelle would like

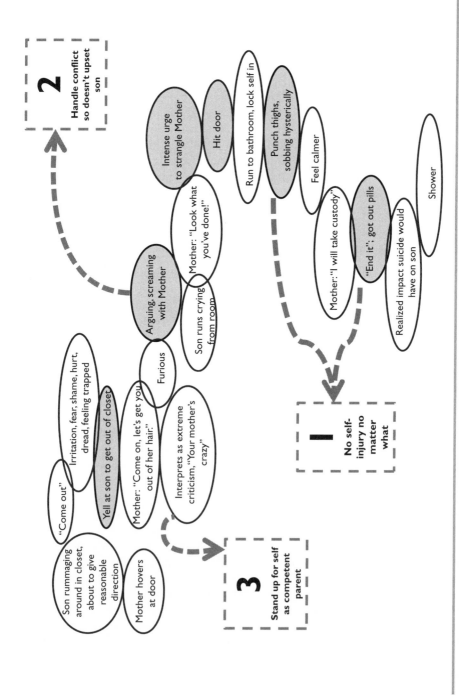

FIGURE 2.3. Places for Jonelle to develop alternative skillful responses.

to be able to effectively stand up to her mother, especially regarding her parenting.

Looking for Patterns across Different Problem Behaviors

As you gather history and preliminary chain analyses on different target behaviors, look for patterns by grouping behavior into classes that function in the same way. For example, let's look for patterns across three chain analyses of primary targets for Samantha as shown in Figure 2.4. These were gathered in the first two sessions of therapy. You'll notice that there's much less detail than in the example with Jonelle; that's because Samantha had a crisis between sessions 1 and 2. Managing the crisis left little time for gathering history. Many clients like Samantha begin therapy amid chaos and crisis management and that disrupts thorough assessment. Nonetheless, you can generate preliminary hypotheses about key controlling variables for primary targets with whatever information you have. Look now at chain analyses of three target behaviors for Samantha: (1) the most recent suicide crisis behavior that prompted her last psychiatric hospital admission; (2) a sequence of therapy-interfering behaviors by client and therapist during and after the first session; and (3) an argument Samantha had with her aunt (that threatens housing and therefore threatens therapy if she moves away). We'll apply the same three sets of concepts (the target hierarchy, biosocial theory, and behavioral theories of change) to look for patterns across target behaviors.

Guided by the target hierarchy, Samantha's therapist prioritized getting a history of suicide attempts and other life-threatening behaviors in the first session. The first chain analysis in Figure 2.4 is of Samantha's overdose on pain medications, a suicide attempt with ambivalent intent to die, that precipitated her last psychiatric hospitalization. The client was living with her parents when she was contacted by a friend, a Marine about to come home on leave from Iraq. Her purging and restricting became more frequent as she wanted "to look good for him." They talked for hours when he got home. He understood completely how bad it feels to have a friend die and to feel responsible. His dark humor expressed empathy without ever having to "talk about it," like a soothing drug. When he left to return to active duty, she was bereft and obsessed that he would be killed. She continued restricting and purging, and stopped taking her pain medication because "it makes me gain weight." She stayed in her room, crying and sleeping and listening to trance music. Her parents were used to her holing up in her room to work on art projects and thought nothing of this. A few days later, in the middle of the night, "things got weird, like they do sometimes." She carved his name in her thigh, fell asleep, then woke, disgusted with herself and with exacerbated back pain from the hunched

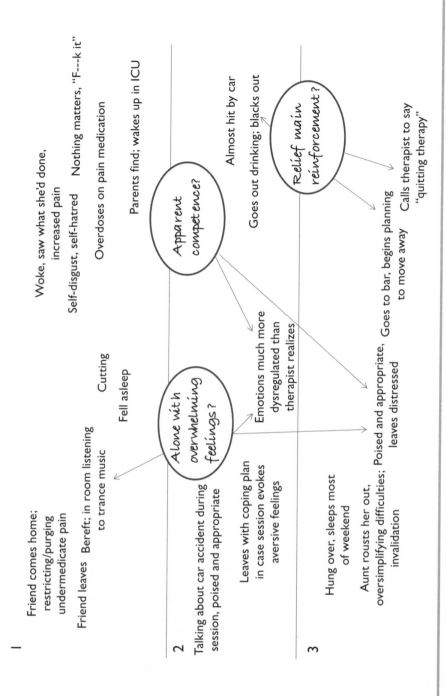

FIGURE 2.4. Comparing three chain analyses of Samantha's important targets.

position she held for hours while cutting. She took pain medication, then took more, and then more, while thinking, "F___k it. Nothing matters." She doesn't remember much after that but said she was found by her parents, and then was taken to a nearby hospital where she ended up in the intensive care unit until she was medically stabilized enough for the psychiatric floor.

The events diagrammed in the figure's second chain analysis began in this first session when the therapist asked Samantha a little about the car accident. Samantha spoke in a poised, strong yet vulnerable, insightful manner that conveyed to the therapist that Samantha was coping remarkably well. The therapist and Samantha made a good plan about how Samantha would manage the predictable increase in feelings that might be evoked by talking with the therapist about the accident. Unbeknown to the therapist, Samantha was extremely dysregulated by the conversation. She left the session so cognitively disorganized that she was almost hit by a car in the parking lot. That night, she went out drinking with friends and drank to the point that she blacked out.

The third chain analysis picks up where the second left off. Samantha slept in all day on Saturday and Sunday. Finally her aunt became so concerned that she rousted her and insisted she "get out of the house and get some fresh air or call your cousin and run out to the community college to see what classes are available." The aunt continued with many problem-solving ideas; Samantha remained pleasant and noncommittal, finally leaving the house acting cheered up for her aunt's benefit. She went to the corner bar and started calling old friends, planning to move. She left the therapist an apologetic message explaining things weren't working out living with her aunt so she'd be moving away and must cancel the next session. (The therapist luckily retrieved her message and reached Samantha before she'd burned any bridges, convincing her to keep their scheduled session the next day.)

What commonalities stand out to you across these different chain analyses? One way to begin is to look for hypotheses from biosocial theory that suggest (1) that disordered behavior may be a consequence of emotion dysregulation or an effort to re-regulate emotion and (2) that invalidation may play a role in maintenance of current difficulties regulating emotion. Look also for the dialectical dilemmas, the secondary behavior patterns described in Chapter 1: emotion vulnerability and self-invalidation, active passivity and apparent competence, and inhibited grieving and unrelenting crisis. Finally, consider what skills deficits, conditioned emotional reactions, contingencies, and cognitive processes or content contribute to Samantha's target behaviors. Figure 2.4 shows the therapist's first pass at identifying each of these common links across target behaviors.

Samantha has many secondary targets. She seldom looks distressed and has a persona of incredible strength. The therapist will want to explicitly orient Samantha to the pattern of apparent competence because it may result in the therapist underestimating distress and suicide risk. Further, Samantha seems caught in a Bermuda triangle of inhibited grieving, unrelenting crises, and emotional vulnerability. Everything reminds her of the car accident; shame and grief become overwhelming; she then impulsively engages in problem behaviors to avoid strong feelings. Even the brief description of the car accident that she gave her therapist at intake felt so overwhelming that it precipitated a crisis. Samantha's secondary targets appear to play a large role in the primary targets of suicide crisis and therapy-interfering behavior.

Samantha's most urgent skills deficits appear to be difficulty tolerating distress without doing something impulsive that actually makes the situation worse. It's not clear yet what contingencies are maintaining Samantha's highest risk behaviors, but her intentional self-injury appears to be maintained by negative reinforcement. It temporarily ends aversive states, such as negative emotions. It does not appear to be maintained by positive reinforcement (i.e., Samantha hides evidence of self-harm and so it does not function to communicate distress to others). Samantha definitely experiences problematic conditioned emotional reactions and emotional dysregulation. The skillful, effective behaviors she does have are often inhibited and disorganized by shame, guilt, unwarranted fears, or other intense or out-of-control emotions. It's not clear yet what cognitive processes or content pose the most problem, but "it doesn't matter," seems to be a recurrent hopeless thought that, for Samantha, precedes a complete passive stance toward living or dying. Samantha's response after discussing the trauma with the therapist provides evidence that Stage 2 exposure work should be postponed until she's stabilized intentional self-injury and disordered eating and has acquired stronger emotion regulation skills.

The therapist created a simplified diagram of Samantha's behavior pattern (see Figure 2.5) and showed it to her in their third session to check whether this accurately captured the key elements of what happens. Although the therapist, at times, takes the lead to highlight, observe, and describe recurrent patterns and comment on implications of behavior, the spirit is one of intentionally fostering that same stance in the client.

As you move through these steps with different target areas and specific problematic behaviors, it is easy to get lost in detail, so focus (and refocus) on what helps you navigate. Go, again and again, for the essence of the problem. It can be helpful to use a one-liner, a label, a metaphor, or a phrase that captures the heart of the problem formulation. Hold it tightly enough so that it can guide you yet hold it lightly enough so that you are

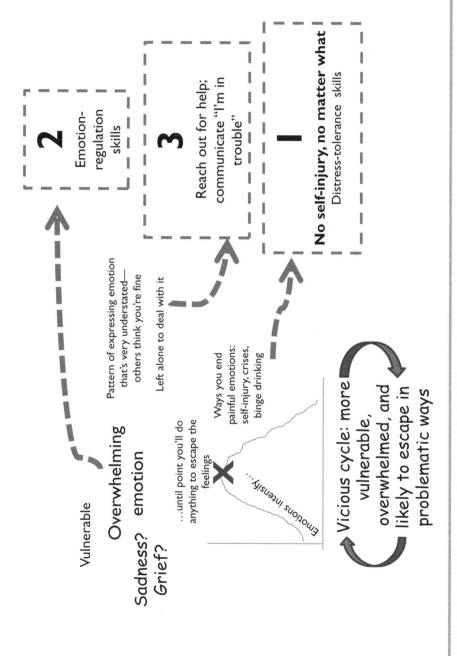

2
Emotion-regulation skills

3
Reach out for help; communicate "I'm in trouble"

1
No self-injury, no matter what
Distress-tolerance skills

Vulnerable

Overwhelming
Sadness? emotion
Grief?

Pattern of expressing emotion that's very understated—others think you're fine

Left alone to deal with it

...until point you'll do anything to escape the feelings

Ways you end painful emotions: self-injury, crises, binge drinking

Emotions intensity...

Vicious cycle: more vulnerable, overwhelmed, and likely to escape in problematic ways

FIGURE 2.5. Simplified pattern diagram, verified with Samantha.

open to influence by new evidence. Strive for "a constantly questioning attitude, a thinking process that incessantly reviews the original hypothesis as it bumps up against the real world. That's what keeps the hypothesis from turning in to a bias that distorts the evidence. It's what leads to original insights and guides the search through a bewildering array of possibly related facts to find what truly matters" (Hart, 2007, p. 21).

The concepts in DBT case formulation that I've been discussing are like orienteering tools. If one doesn't work, pick up another until the picture of controlling variables become clear, or at least clear enough to take the next step.

STEP 3: USE TASK ANALYSIS TO GENERATE MINI-TREATMENT PLANS FOR KEY COMMON LINKS

A task analysis describes the step-by-step behavioral sequence required to get from the client's current capability and circumstance to the desired behavior or outcome. You and the client may conduct a spontaneous task analysis in the flow of conversation or may do it in a more deliberate way. The question you ask is, "What would be a more effective response in this circumstance?" Identify this replacement behavior for each target behavior and the most common dysfunctional links. Next, figure out *exactly* what the client must do to engage in the replacement behavior. Then create "mini"-treatment plans to help the client move from old behaviors to new ones at key junctures.

For these mini-treatment plans, draw strategies from three pools. First, consider replacing dysfunctional links with DBT skills. Second, look to the research literature on treatment and normal psychology for replacement behaviors. Finally, consider personal experience. How exactly did you or others you know solve a similar problem? The key with task analysis is to be sure that the replacement behavior you select actually works for the client's circumstance. For example, when a person is highly dysregulated, it is nearly impossible to do skills that require complicated thinking. In that circumstance, the step-by-step task analysis should begin with strategies that target emotion regulation before a skill that requires the client to already be regulated, such as an interpersonal effectiveness skill. Finding situation-specific solutions can be an incredible challenge. For example, how do *you*, in the midst of extreme emotional arousal and inadequate interpersonal support, inhibit impulsive actions and instead do what is effective for that moment? This aspect of task analysis calls for using empathy in a way that is like spatial awareness. It is as if someone calls you on the phone for directions but is unsure where he is or how his location relates to where he wants to go. If you know the area well, you can describe the landmarks to get his confirmation that he's where you think he is; then you can describe exactly how to proceed. Step by step, exactly how does he get from here to there? At times a client cannot or will not articulate what is happening, which requires the therapist to have a highly refined ability to locate the client. For example, Samantha's therapist rapidly learned to read highly subtle cues that indicated Samantha was more dysregulated than was apparent. She then knew to move Samantha to activities such as using a balance board and holding ice, which help re-regulate emotion, before she left the session.

For example, the therapist and Jonelle did a task analysis of exactly how Jonelle would prefer to handle moments when her mother hovered, ready to criticize Jonelle's parenting. They began by imagining an outcome and set of interactions that Jonelle would feel proud of. She wished she could say to her mother: "Please leave; I don't want your help parenting right now. He minds just fine when we have the space to do it our way." Then Jonelle and the therapist went step by step to determine how Jonelle could get from where she is to the responses she'd prefer. Jonelle would need the ability to recognize when she needs to assert herself. Their assessment showed Jonelle did not have this ability, so self-monitoring was used to increase awareness. She needed to have the interpersonal skills to obtain her objective, while maintaining the relationship and her self-respect. Jonelle knew how to act to avoid conflict, but not how to achieve her objective and keep her self-respect. As the therapist and Jonelle role-played various ways Jonelle might observe her limit with her mother, it became apparent that Jonelle believed she had forfeited any rights to speak up. She felt great shame about her failings as a mother. Shame even came up when the therapist, role-playing her mother, made an unreasonable request; Jonelle became completely dysregulated and capitulated. Therefore, another important step of the task was to help Jonelle regulate shame. Cognitive restructuring was also used to help her actually believe she had the right to assert herself. She also needed the ability to regulate her anger when her mother verbally attacked and criticized her. Jonelle had skills and used them at work, but did not use them in intimate relationships. As she and her therapist further assessed Jonelle's skills, it became clear that when her mother hurt her feelings, it was followed quickly by anger and judgmental thoughts. Following her mother's hurtful words, Jonelle would think, "She shouldn't be like that! Of all people, she should understand and support me!" Therefore, another piece of the task was to help Jonelle radically accept that, for many reasons, her mother often was critical and unsupportive. The therapist's mini-treatment plans for each of Jonelle's specific problems add up to make the full treatment plan that includes:

- Solution generation to identify needs, wants, and values with respect to conflict with her mother.
- Self-monitoring (to recognize when she needs to be assertive) with her mother.
- Skills training (for emotion regulation of shame and anger, interpersonal effectiveness, and radical acceptance).
- Imaginal exposure (to reduce the conditioned shame response to criticism).
- Cognitive modification (of beliefs about asserting herself).

Acting skillfully is no simple proposition. Many of us have the ability to patiently redirect a child until he or she stops misbehaving. However, when critical parents or in-laws are watching our child disobey our instructions, it is a much more difficult situation. Can we then patiently redirect the child, ignoring or assertively blocking the other adult's undermining statements? Or when we become too frustrated to be effective, can we let in their help? We may have the component abilities such as knowing what to say to our child, being able to regulate our frustration and embarrassment, being able to accurately read whether the other adult is judging us, being open and nondefensive, and so on, but putting it all together under pressure is what makes for a skillful response. By analogy, in the privacy of a weekday morning at a nearby basketball court, I can shoot a net-swishing free throw. But that is different from being able to execute it in a game and different still from being able to do it in the last seconds of a championship game. DBT treatment plans therefore emphasize not only skills training but skills strengthening and generalization to progressively more difficult situations like those faced in daily life, that is, not just practice, but practice in all relevant contexts. Behavioral rehearsal is essential and emphasized in all DBT treatment plans.

Across situations, clients experience recurring problems when they try to adopt more functional behavior. When you see these recurring obstacles, return to the four factors from behavior therapy to guide assessment of likely controlling variables. Ask:

1. What are the skills deficits?
2. What emotional reactions interfere with more skillful responses?
3. Which contingencies are problematic?
4. What cognitions or cognitive processes interfere with more skillful responses?

For example, Samantha's pattern across problems highlighted how often apparent competence interfered with getting the help she needed. The immediate therapy task was to help Samantha tolerate distress without making things worse. But distress so dysregulated Samantha that her brain simply wouldn't function. She needed more help and yet she was ashamed to ask for help. She was afraid of the devastating disappointment she would feel if the therapist was unavailable when needed, and extremely scared to open up and then be left alone with overwhelming feelings. But you'd never know this from looking at her. Even while expressing distress her poise and apparent competence constantly led others to assume no help was needed. To address the problem, the therapist and Samantha began to implement contingency management strategies along with behavioral rehearsal: Samantha was to call every day at a pre-specified time for 2 weeks to practice, whether she needed help or not. Her task was to accurately express (as best she could) what her current emotions were. The therapist, alerted to the helpfulness of Samantha's Marine friend's banter, kept the calls light but deeply empathic as she coached use of distress tolerance skills.

Mini-plans to treat specific problems and mechanisms add up to make the full treatment plan. You use the tools of chain analysis and task analysis to see what paths lead to important target behaviors, what on the paths needs to change, and what might get in the way of change. Perhaps most importantly, you learn what is common across time and across problem areas. This allows you to focus on changing those processes that will affect multiple targets.

Once you can see recurrent patterns, then you can more quickly locate yourself and your client on the chain of events and more quickly see where to work at any given moment. It is as if you, the therapist, were a quality control inspector examining lengths of chain for problems with individual links. As you hear about your client's life and observe what happens in session, your priorities are to pick up those lengths of the behavior chain that end with intentional self-injury, therapy-interfering behavior, or behavior interfering with the client's quality of life.

Usually there is no shortage of problematic behavior. The struggle is to choose where to intervene and how to sustain intervention in the face of slow change and extreme distress. Choosing well means to "pick up the correct length of chain" that leads to primary treatment targets (intentional self-injury, therapy-interfering behavior, and behavior interfering with the client's quality of life). You work on change wherever the client happens to be on that chain. When the client reports that he or she is now experiencing vulnerability factors that in the past led to problem behaviors, treat those vulnerability factors. When a client is at imminent risk for suicide, however, the links that most need inspection and correction are those associated with immediate danger. In essence, the therapist goes over the edge, toolkit in hand, and fixes each link within reach during the therapy hour, preferably in a manner that teaches the client to fix links for the rest of the week between sessions. When the client is further from the edge, the therapist can "inspect and repair" those links that occur earlier in the chain. Visually diagramming these pathways can be very helpful for both clients and therapists, so that they together identify how to move away from problematic responses and toward adaptive responses. Prioritize how to avoid at all costs (1) engaging in life-threatening behavior, (2) catching the patterns early when the client is still more regulated and capable, and (3) finding alternatives to common links across problems.

Throughout the process of formulating and treatment planning, continually summarize, paraphrase, and check things out with the client. Be transparent, collaborative, and psychoeducational (as much as is useful to the particular client) as you refine, verify, or discard hypotheses. Repeat this process to look for the controlling variables for each important problem behavior.

And throughout the process, it's important to maintain a dialectical thinking style, a stance that keeps your mind agile and flexible. From a dialectical stance, therefore, feeling stuck or polarized becomes a useful cue, a reminder that you've temporarily forgotten the nature of reality and taken the bit you happen to hold in your hand as the whole, absolute truth. Tension, confusion, and polarity between the client and therapist and among team members about how to best understand and treat problems are expected—even welcomed—and used as cues to open up to look for what is valid in opposing views.

The conversational or thinking style of dialectical assessment can feel a lot like pushing one of those old-fashioned red-and-white balls used as fishing bobbers under the water with the tip of your finger. The pointed tension in a conversation or line of thought creates a countertension in the same way that holding a bobber under the water does. The pressure from the point of contact makes the bobber roll to pop up in a different place. To illustrate, say a client felt immediate emotional relief when she burnt her arms with cigarettes and was reluctant to give it up. As the therapist assessed the factors that led to a recent incident, the client nonchalantly said, "The burn really wasn't that bad this time." The therapist responded to accentuate the inherent contradictions in the client's responses:

THERAPIST: So what you're saying is that if you saw a person in a lot of emotional pain, say your little niece, and she was feeling as badly as you were the night you burned your arm—she was feeling as devastated by disappointment as you were that night—you'd burn her arm with a cigarette to help her feel better.

CLIENT: No, I wouldn't.

THERAPIST: Why not?

CLIENT: I just wouldn't.

THERAPIST: I believe you wouldn't, but why not?

CLIENT: I'd comfort her or do something else to help her feel better.

THERAPIST: But what if she was inconsolable—nothing you did made her feel better? Besides, you wouldn't burn her that badly.

CLIENT: I just wouldn't do it. It's not right. I'd do something, but not that.

THERAPIST: That's interesting, don't you think?

The client simultaneously believes that one should not burn someone under any circumstances and that burning herself to get relief is no big deal. This style of dialectically assessing "how do these go together for you" yielded important information about the client's values (similar to building discrepancy in motivational interviewing). A dialectical stance prioritizes exploring such inconsistencies among the client's own actions, beliefs, and values as well as the therapist's inconsistencies. Such exploration in itself may prompt change as the dialectically informed dialogue focuses on helping clients and therapists reach a viewpoint that is more whole and internally consistent.

When confused, polarized, or stuck, you assess what's left out and what's valid in each position so that case formulation and treatment planning are a series of dialogues that lead to synthesis rather than rigid reasoning from immutable facts. All assessment should promote contact with and dialogue about what interferes with clients having the life that they want. Any solution or intervention must take into account the multiple valid points of the dialogue in order to be effective. Attention is not on the client alone, but rather the relationships among the client, the client's community, the therapist, and the therapist's community.

A PRETREATMENT CONVERSATION: MANNY

The rest of this chapter is an extended example of dialogue from an initial pretreatment session. It illustrates how a therapist uses target hierarchies to prioritize assessment and looks for variables that may be controlling target behaviors, particularly Stage 1 life-threatening and therapy-interfering behaviors. However, the gathering of this information, such as in an informal chain analysis, is a change strategy that can set off emotion dysregulation in the client. Therefore, the therapist dialectically balances change with acceptance strategies such as validation throughout the interaction to help the client re-regulate and stay present in the conversation.

At the same time, the therapist is also assessing the priorities of the pretreatment stage. Will client and therapist be able to agree on the goals and methods of therapy? What barriers, if any, are there? Is there sufficient client commitment to treatment? A key task is for the therapist to orient the client to therapy while also working to build client motivation and commitment. Many times clients feel reluctant to make needed changes. They may hesitate, feel ambivalent, or downright refuse to agree to components of therapy that you believe are needed. This is particularly true at pretreatment but may occur in big and small ways throughout the course of therapy. The therapist must again and again ensure that the treatment methods and plan link directly and vividly to the client's ultimate goals. Identifying those goals is an important task of the initial sessions. Linehan (1993a) outlined a number of commitment strategies that strengthen the client's commitment to change. For example, the therapist in the dialogue that follows uses the "foot-in-the-door" strategy to describe generally and favorably the link between the client's goals and wishes and treatment. Later in the session, the therapist emphasizes the client's freedom to choose not to enter DBT while at the same time highlighting the client's lack of real alternatives so that the client can reckon for herself what change will involve and the costs of the status quo if she doesn't change. The foundation of these strategies needs to be flexibility and an honest respect for the client's choices and goals.

At these moments, when the client is ambivalent, you formulate the problem and plan treatment by balancing opposing positions and working to find genuine syntheses. You balance the client's needs, goals, and preferences with your own professional and personal limits to reach a true workable agreement for therapy. You use the target hierarchy to guide chain analyses and weave DBT's core strategies (change, validation, and dialectical strategies) to assess and treat the highest priority target.

In the dialogue that follows, the therapist has come to a local inpatient unit to meet with the client as a condition of her discharge. The client, Manny, has had very serious nonsuicidal self-injury as well as multiple high-risk suicide attempts. She's had multiple therapies, none of which she viewed as helpful in the end, and is hopeless. In her lifetime she's been given diagnoses of chronic PTSD, bipolar not otherwise specified (NOS), atypical psychotic, BPD, and intermittent explosive disorder. Manny's current hospitalization occurred after an overdose precipitated by a falling out with her prior therapist who is refusing to resume Manny's care. The dialogue has been edited, with detailed history gathering omitted. The conversation begins after a few preliminaries.

THERAPIST: You mentioned on the phone that you had mixed feelings about whether to try therapy again. If you were going to get into therapy again, what would you want my help with?

MANNY: I don't really know. Everybody's been telling me that DBT, whatever that is, is the thing for me, so that's why I agreed to meet with you.

THERAPIST: Hmm.

MANNY: But therapy in general has not worked for me.

THERAPIST: Mm hmm. So, people have a lot of opinions about you needing to get into therapy, but you're not sure what help therapy can offer. I'm happy to tell you more about how we would work if we decide to work together and use DBT (*warm, responsive style and emphasis on validation of the client's perspective*), but I guess I'd like to hear more about what you mean that therapy has not worked for you.

MANNY: I'm surprised you are even considering being my therapist. I didn't think anyone would take me, given Dr. Jones kicked me out.

THERAPIST: (*Follows the conversational flow and takes the opportunity to assess therapy-interfering behavior of Manny and her former therapist.*) So, what happened with your former therapist that she "kicked you out"? (*Assesses therapy-interfering behavior, dialectical stance means assuming both likely contributed.*)

MANNY: Well, I had been doing better in some ways, and then I went downhill and she couldn't take it anymore.

THERAPIST: What pushed her over the edge? (*Uses warm, matter-of-fact tone, communicates that the therapist has no judgment or preconception that Manny was the problem; it could have been that the former therapist was too fragile.*)

MANNY: I started hurting myself again, and then I took an overdose after I told her that I had gotten rid of the pills.

THERAPIST: (*Hearing an opportunity to assess the highest-priority target, the suicide attempt, therapist refines focus of the assessment.*) So, you were doing better, then somehow you went back to the old behavior of hurting yourself, then somewhere in there you started hoarding pills but not telling your therapist . . . ?

MANNY: Yeah, I was going back to school and I got a work-study job in the library but this guy in one of my classes started stalking me, he started to hang out in the parking lot, and be there at closing and then I ended up just quitting everything.

THERAPIST: You must've been so disappointed! And scared . . .

MANNY: Yeah, I talked to the police, but they said they couldn't do anything (*uses total blasé voice*) so I ended up trying to get my mom to help with money so I could quit at the library but she wouldn't help and . . .

THERAPIST: (*Gently interrupts.*) You know, as you're talking you sound very matter-of-fact, almost casual, but I get the sense that this was a tremendous setback for you . . . (*Notes discrepancy between content and emotional expression and moves to assessing for apparent competence and difficulties in accurately expressing or experiencing emotion. Hypothesizes that this may be a factor that interfered with prior therapy, making it hard for the therapist to read how distressed the client was.*)

MANNY: Yeah, I was actually doing good that quarter.

THERAPIST: So, that must have made it even more painful, or disappointing?

MANNY: Yes.

THERAPIST: Yes, you know your voice tone about all this, the way you are saying it, it sounds like you had a problem finding a parking space. (*Exactly replicates Manny's breezy tone.*) "Yeah, you know, I was having the best quarter ever, really getting my life together and then this guy stalked me, and the police couldn't help, my mom wouldn't help, so I lost it all." (*Uses an irreverent communication style to prompt change while validating difficulty.*)

MANNY: (*Laughs.*)

THERAPIST: I could see mistaking your tone of voice to mean this is not important to you . . . but it was a huge setback, wasn't it?

MANNY: Yes. (*Her eye contact conveys that the therapist has understood exactly and Manny feels relieved.*)

THERAPIST: (*Files away apparent competence as hypothesis that might be relevant but due to time constraints wants to get more detail on higher-order targets.*) There's this huge setback with school, and when did you start harming yourself again? (*Uses target hierarchy to keep priority on identifying what leads to intentional self-injury, beginning high-level chain analysis.*)

MANNY: When my mom said she wouldn't help, I knew I had to drop out, and we were on the phone.

THERAPIST: You and your mom?

MANNY: No, me and my therapist. I was really crazy inside, and she called me back, and then she talked me into making a cup of tea, and then I just got so mad I poured the water over my hand.

THERAPIST: While she was still on the phone with you?

MANNY: No. I hung up on her. Then I just did it. Then I saw her the next day, and I had had to go to the emergency room because I had burned myself so bad and had all these bandages on my hand and she's like, "What happened?" and I'm like, "Well, the tea didn't really help."

THERAPIST: Hmm. That sounds like you were really mad at her . . .

(Difficulty regulating anger? Problems with assertiveness? Therapist's failure to recognize extent of client's difficulties or Manny's deficit in communicating? Stimulus control problem whenever means to self-harm are available, as Manny can't inhibit behavior?)

MANNY: I was mad at everybody. I broke my hand when I hit a wall earlier that week, I almost got into a fight waiting for my bus, I was totally out of control.

THERAPIST: Yeah, I see what you're saying. Is that something that happens a lot? *(OK, difficulty regulating anger?)*

MANNY: What, getting that mad and out of control?

THERAPIST: Yeah.

MANNY: I, I just screwed it all up. *(Shows big shift in affect.)*

THERAPIST: *(Files away need to come back and assess anger further, but noticing that Manny seems to feel either shame or perhaps sadness about loss of last therapist. Therapist is sensitive to the possibility that perhaps now in-session dysregulation may be occurring, that maybe asking about frequency felt invalidating. Therapist stays on chain that led to overdose but thinks increasing validation might be useful.)*

   (Gentle but matter-of-fact tone.) Yeah, that kind of thing can really strain a relationship. You really wish things had gone differently and feel a lot of regret, it looks like . . . *(Validates emotion and reads Manny's adaptive and positive intent.)*

MANNY: *(Silently nods.)*

THERAPIST: *(Has choice of either assessing for emotional dysregulation further and perhaps treating it a bit or continuing with assessment of past suicide attempt. Uses matter-of-fact nonjudgmental voice tone to assist Manny in regulating emotion and in continuing with conversation without further heightening emotional experience.)* I am glad you're telling me about how hard this was. So, you lost school and then that week you were really angry, kind of out of control, then you burn your hand, and then you're talking about it with your therapist and then what happened?

MANNY: She said she wasn't going to work with me if I keep doing that, she could transfer me, but she'd had it.

THERAPIST: You sound like this came as a surprise.

MANNY: I could tell she was kind of freaked out over the summer when I came in with my arms all cut up, but . . . she understands I get to the point where I can't take it and then I hurt myself. *(Manny's manner of phrasing this raises hypothesis that having cuts visible to the therapist may have been communication about how much misery she was experiencing and therapist notes need to come back and further assess whether self-injury is maintained by communicating to others. Manny also highlights a potential deficit in distress tolerance skills ["get to the point where I can't take it"]. However, now the therapist prioritizes understanding the suicide attempt.)* But she said that she wasn't willing to work with me if I was going to act out at her in that way.

THERAPIST: So, it was really past her limit to have you hurt yourself right after she tried to help.

MANNY: Yeah, but it wasn't about her, I was getting so out of control I needed to calm down . . . I was just so . . . I just couldn't stand it, so I just did it, it was stupid, but I did it.

THERAPIST: So, you were desperate for relief, she tried to help, even though it wasn't about her . . . something about the call or getting off the call . . . Something in there seems to have actually made things worse, and then you scalded your hand?

MANNY: Yeah.

THERAPIST: And then—what—you just kind of showed up with the bandages and . . . ?

MANNY: Yeah, I almost didn't go, I knew she'd take it bad. It was a crappy, stupid thing to do.

THERAPIST: Yeah, not a shining moment to say "the tea didn't work," yeah. Sounds like a really difficult conversation. This might be a place we work together, you know—how to help you have these really painful emotions somehow without ending up doing things that you later so regret. Would that feel right to you? *(Gently begins change-oriented work of building commitment.)*

MANNY: Yeah, I just get so out of control, and screw everything up, it's been that way my whole life.

THERAPIST: Yeah, I can feel how much you don't want that to happen. You asked about DBT earlier, and one part of it is exactly for what we're talking about here. A lot of people who have very intense emotions never get to learn how to handle overwhelming emotions. One of the skill modules is exactly for this kind of moment you're describing, you learn how to tolerate distress so you don't do things you regret later. Right now all you can do is white-knuckle it—you don't have enough options to help when emotions get so overwhelming.

MANNY: Yeah.

THERAPIST: OK, so she said, "Look, I can't work with you if you do this," and then what'd you say? *(Again the therapist attempts to minimally treat shame by increasing tolerance for it even amid the higher-priority task of assessing the chain leading to the suicide attempt. The therapist's voice tone is matter of fact, conveying complete acceptance without judgment and yet not shying away from the fact that Manny views her own behavior as unacceptable.)*

MANNY: (*Very solemn, as if saying a final good-bye.*) I said I really appreciated everything she'd done for me, she'd been a great therapist, and I was really sorry I screwed up therapy just like everything else.

THERAPIST: Hmm, that doesn't sound good. (*Reads the finality and guesses increased suicide ideation.*)

MANNY: And then I went home and took an overdose.

THERAPIST: So, in the conversation, somewhere in there, you decided to kill yourself?

MANNY: You know, sometimes, you have to face that it's your own fault, no one's doing it to you, and you should stop making everyone else suffer, you know? Just end it.

THERAPIST: So, somewhere in the conversation you started thinking like that, condemning yourself?

MANNY: Yeah.

THERAPIST: . . . Shame at how you'd handled things, blaming yourself for all your problems. Almost sounds like really strong self-hatred, yes?

MANNY: (*Nods.*)

THERAPIST: . . . Yes, that's a dark, dark place. So, you need some help with that place, maybe in therapy . . . and then you took an overdose?

MANNY: Yes.

THERAPIST: What exactly did you take? (*Therapist redacts detailed suicide risk assessment history here.*) Let me say back to you what I understand so far to see if I get it, ok? The root of things that led up to you trying to kill yourself started when you lost everything, then couldn't get help, and then you started to get out of control, angry, doing things you regret, and the emotions got so intense you started going back to old behaviors to cope . . . yes?

MANNY: Yes.

THERAPIST: And then somehow when things get that hard, and you aren't getting help you need, somehow you start hating yourself for being a burden, for having all these problems, and try to kill yourself, kind of to take yourself out of misery and spare other people the misery too . . . ?

MANNY: Yes.

THERAPIST: Then you end up here against your will, and people are wanting you to start DBT . . . am I getting it?

MANNY: Yeah, that's it. You got it.

THERAPIST: Well, let me tell you what I think I might offer. But let me say, first, that I only do voluntary treatment, OK, I only work with people when we both think it's a good idea and have agreed to exactly how we're going to work together. That's what I see us doing now— you telling me how things go for you, me telling you if I think working together we could help them go different and more like you want. I'd want to talk more about what you want, but if after that, we both feel like we're a good team together and we can do the work you want to do, then we'll make a formal commitment about how long we're agreeing to work together, how we'll handle any problems that come up between us, things like that. I can already tell I like you, which is a big thing for me, how are you feeling? Comfortable talking or . . . ?

MANNY: Yeah, I am kind of surprised I'm talking so much, I don't usually do that . . .

THERAPIST: OK, I feel that, that's neat and a good start for us. Let me tell you the ideas I have so far to see if they fit for you and seem worth trying. I work mostly with people who have very intense emotions who through no fault of their own never learned ways to work with emotions. They get trapped and can't get life problems solved and then emotion gets out of control and people find that harming themselves gives relief, it makes the emotion stop, like you said earlier that cutting makes you feel calm.

MANNY: Right.

THERAPIST: So, the therapy I offer is for people who have intense emotions and helps them learn other ways to help themselves other than self-injury. But for a lot of people giving up self-injury is hard. Have you ever tried to stop before?

MANNY: Yes, I try not to do it, but sometimes it's the only thing that helps.

THERAPIST: Yeah. (*Pauses.*)

MANNY: I mean I know it's messed up, but sometimes it's cut or kill myself, you know?

THERAPIST: Yeah. A lot of people feel like that when they start our program . . . where they feel like if they can't relieve the tension, they get more suicidal.

MANNY: Exactly.

THERAPIST: Right. So what's the longest you've ever gone?

MANNY: I guess I went almost a year one time, and just before all this stuff happened this summer and fall . . . I guess it'd been 4 months I was doing better.

THERAPIST: Wow. It almost makes me cry to think of how hard that time was for you. Wow. OK, so you know next time we meet, if you decide you want to meet again, we might want to talk about what you already know about how to stop but I guess, right now, the more important question for us is, all things being equal, would you rather have a different way of helping yourself with these intense emotions and life problems? I mean, are you attached to being a cutter or anything? (*Uses foot-in-the-door to begin building commitment to therapy.*)

MANNY: What do you mean?

THERAPIST: I mean like for some people, it's part of their identity, who they are.

MANNY: No, it's not like that, it's just I can't stand it.

THERAPIST: Right. I guess based on what you've told me, my question to you is, it seems like what you really need is a solution where when your life is falling apart—you know, truly bad things are happening—one thing you need is more help with the actual problems like money for school, getting safe—you know, those were real problems and more help would've been good. And then the second thing you need is there are times when the emotional pain gets where you can't stand it, and I'm wondering if we worked together could we work on how, when there is this overwhelming emotional pain, for you to have ways to help yourself other than cutting? How would it fit for you to work on that?

MANNY: That's just not going to happen, you know, I've tried a lot of therapy, it just never goes well.

THERAPIST: Yeah, I need to understand that more . . . because I know for me, I wouldn't want you to try something you know and get disappointed again . . . you've tried a lot of therapy. (*Accepts Manny's legitimate worry while continuing to strengthen commitment to change.*)

MANNY: Yeah.

THERAPIST: Yeah. (*Long pause.*) I'd really want us to talk more about that so we're both sure our therapy would get you where you want to go. One place I would propose we start is using your urges to harm yourself, especially thoughts of killing yourself, as our indicator light of where things are most difficult—we would really work to help you with the real life problems that make you want to be dead and help you have more options with overwhelming emotions. Do you know much about learning theory?

MANNY: No.

THERAPIST: OK, so let me just draw this on the whiteboard, OK? Here's emotion intensity and here's time. When something happens to make an emotion fire, it goes up like this. OK, for some people it's slow to set off and only goes up some and then pretty quickly comes down. But for some people it's more like this—it fires and then up here it is completely unbearable and a person will do anything to escape. This is where I think you say, "I can't take it."

MANNY: Yeah, I can't.

THERAPIST: But the problem is that if you escape here at the most intense point, what does your brain learn?

MANNY: What?

THERAPIST: Think about your brain like a kid that really wants something and is escalating "Give me escape!!" like a kid would scream "I want candy!" Say, you then give it escape, what happens the next time your brain is in the candy store, so to speak?

MANNY: It has an even worse tantrum—this is just like my niece, who is 3.

THERAPIST: Right, and then you give in eventually because she is screaming so loudly. You escape the discomfort of her screaming. So, how about the next time, how high does the emotion go if you try to hold off escaping? . . .

MANNY: As high as it needs to to get me to give in.

THERAPIST: Right. *That's* the problem with self-injury as a solution. If you want emotions to come down . . . it works in the moment, but it makes it worse and worse in future situations. That make sense?

MANNY: So I get relief when I cut, but then if I hold out trying not to cut then my emotions keep going up and up and eventually I give in . . .

THERAPIST: Right. So, if you were going to help your niece having an out-of-control emotion, would you give in or what would be your treatment?

MANNY: No. I would never give in . . . I mean eventually she'd learn not to have tantrums if I didn't give in.

THERAPIST: Yeah. That's in essence what I would propose we do. If we decide to work together, we would look at all the circumstances and life problems that set off these unbearable emotions and then we'd do several things at once to help. First is that you don't have enough options in these moments where things are hardest and most overwhelming. So, I mentioned the skills training earlier, and if we start soon, then I would love for you to join the group of Gary and Kristen, because they are hilarious, great teachers, and really genuine as people, and I think you might like them. (*Continues change-oriented commitment work.*) You'd learn a lot of skills so you'd have a lot more help in these hardest moments. Another thing I'd suggest is that you and I work very, very hard and closely together, and I would be available to you on the phone to help in real time to offer ideas and help you through. Because it is unbelievably hard to change intentional self-injury because it works, it ends the emotional pain. But just like you said with your niece, when your brain screams it can't take it, what we'd do is stay close and ride these through so that under no circumstances would you give in when your brain screams it has to escape. . . . It'll be some white-knuckling at first, and then over time you'll have more skills and it'll get easier. (*Pauses.*) So, it'll look like this over time . . .

MANNY: What do you mean no escape?

THERAPIST: When I say no escape, I mean that I think we should agree to take these escape strategies like cutting and attempting suicide completely off the table for a period of time while you learn new ways to work with emotional pain. I mean, you've tried other therapies where you got support and kept using your escape strategies and you were just describing how that's not worked . . . (*Continues to accept Manny's legitimate worries to strengthen commitment to change.*)

MANNY: Yeah. (*Both are silent, looking at the whiteboard together.*) So you're saying I would have to not do any of these escapes . . .

THERAPIST: Actually, I'm not saying you "have to" do anything. Like I said, I only work with people where we both really agree about what we're doing (*emphasizes freedom to choose*) . . . I think more what I'm saying is look, here's my understanding of how brains work. If you want things to go differently, you have to find some way other than escape. Support plus occasional escape, you've tried. You are of course free to try that some more . . . (*says with a light tone and smile that Manny shares*), no, seriously, this way of not escaping is really, really hard, and I bet the social workers could help find some other options besides me, so I really mean it about you choosing if you want to go down this path. But if we work together, then I think, especially seeing now some of the strengths you have and this initial feel of how easy it is for us to talk, I think if we took this escape stuff off the table and really worked our rear ends off, I think in 4–6 months you'd have learned to manage these intense moments in a way you feel good about, and in a year we could really make more of a life you want . . . It'd be really hard, you know, maybe harder than anything you've ever done in your life . . . (*Long pause. The therapist internally shifts fully away from change and deeply into appreciating the magnitude of pain in Manny's life, following her breathing.*)

MANNY: OK. (*Both are silent.*) . . . Let me think about it . . . It's a big commitment . . .

THERAPIST: Yeah. For the kind of payoff you want, I'm thinking that's what's needed . . . yeah . . . and I think it's good to really think about it, because it is really hard to give up escape and find a different way . . . We're right at the end of our meeting time . . . I guess, let me say, I've learned enough to feel interested in continuing the conversation, I have a good feeling about working together, and really it's up to you at this point whether we should meet again . . .

MANNY: Let me, let me think a bit.

THERAPIST: Sure. (*Warm, easy manner.*) Sure. If I were you, I'd need time to think, too, that's totally fine. The social worker said you're here for 2 more days, that right?

MANNY: Yes.

THERAPIST: OK, well, I'm back on this side of town late afternoon tomorrow, so if you have questions or whatever, that would be a good time for me to meet. Just call and let me know if you want to meet again. Here's my cell phone number—that's by far the best way to reach me. (*Hands Manny a card with a handwritten note.*) OK (*stands, reaches to shake hands, very warm*), I'll wait to hear, and of course now knowing that I like you I'm hoping you want to continue the conversation but of course it's a big decision. . . . Do you want to walk me out?

MANNY: Yeah.

This example shows how the concepts discussed in this chapter are used to guide initial interactions. By using the target hierarchy, biosocial theory, and secondary targets, and then adding behavioral theories of change, the therapist assessed the problems prompting Manny's referral. Figure 2.6 and Table 2.2 begin to organize the information gleaned so far. Figure 2.6 shows the therapist's attempt to capture the chain and the initial further assessment questions in a rough fashion soon after the first contact. Table 2.2 is organized according to the Stage 1 priority target hierarchy and further elaborates the therapist's "notes to self" that will direct the next round of assessment questions. Therapists will differ in the ways that help them remember controlling variables and I've included these rough early representations of a therapist's thinking to encourage you to experiment, even with very rough sketches, and to help you understand

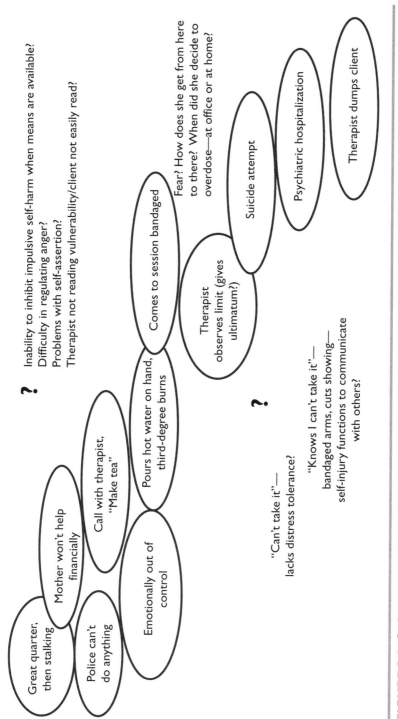

FIGURE 2.6. Preliminary visual notes for Manny's case formulation and treatment plan.

TABLE 2.2. **Therapist Notes by Target Area**

Pretreatment

- Need to understand still what Manny wants, what are we working toward—back to school? What?
- My limits: need to come to agreement about Manny's hoarding medications/not disclosing honestly.

Life-threatening

- Overdose, hoarding medications, failing to tell therapist/lying to therapist about this? When did she start hoarding meds? When exactly did she decide to take the overdose? What does she have now? What set off her not disclosing her hoarding of medications—how can we make sure this goes differently for us?
- Pour scalding water, third-degree burns: impulsive? Can she control impulses in the presence of means of self-harm? What exactly was going on in the phone call that precipitated this event?
- Cuts visible to the therapist—does her self-injury function to communicate to others?
- How bad is "getting out of control"—almost getting into a fight at bus stop? Risk of her getting hurt or hurting others?
- "It's your own fault," "stop making others suffer," intense shame—assess further to determine if common across suicidal behavior and nonsuicidal self-injury.

Therapy-interfering

- Prior therapist unwilling to resume therapy after suicide attempt. Per client, after therapist observed limit ("I won't keep working with you if you act out this way after I try to help"). Client scalded hand, requiring medical attention, after client hung up on therapist during phone call. "Therapist couldn't take (self-injury) anymore." Client says she got rid of pills, but in fact she was hoarding them and took an overdose. Need more detail—client OK if she and I get specifics of what went wrong so we don't repeat?
- Directly observed that client's manner of speaking about distress was incongruent with actual distress she experiences. Somehow, while getting help, interactions go terribly wrong—why?

Quality of life

- Difficulty with anger? Shame?
- See if there's a good diagnostic workup in inpatient chart or whether one could be done prior to discharge.

Skills deficits

- Definitely has distress tolerance difficulties.
- Somehow unable to get help she needs from mom, police, and past therapist—why?

the common patterns of controlling variables for your clients. The therapist in this case wonders if one major context associated with suicidal behavior for this client is when she is unable to elicit appropriate help from others, perhaps due to the combination of her own interpersonal skills deficits and the secondary target of apparent competence, and/or perhaps due to the overwhelming action urge of intense shame that keeps her silent. She also has questions about the best way to conceptualize actions like pouring boiling water over her hand. The therapist suspects that self-injury serves more than one function. It is likely an impulsive escape from distress and so improving distress tolerance skills will be needed. However, given the client's report that her past therapist was upset at seeing evidence of self-injury, the therapist will also want to assess whether self-injury serves to communicate distress. The therapist in the next session will be particularly focused on understanding what led the client to fail to disclose that she was hoarding medication, to understand the controlling variables of that important link in the chain to suicidal behavior. You may have found while reading the transcript that different questions and hypotheses came up for you than did for the therapist. That's to be expected and even hoped for in DBT because divergent views may more rapidly lead to useful understanding of the client's problems and the best way to approach them. This excerpt also illustrates a common pretreatment interaction, giving a first glimpse of how the therapist blends DBT's core strategies to assess, orient, and build commitment to change. We turn now to show in detail the change-oriented behavioral strategies (Chapter 3), acceptance-oriented validation strategies (Chapter 4), and dialectical strategies (Chapter 5).

THREE

Change Strategies

During these brief days that you have strength,
be quick and spare no effort of your wings.
                                                    —RUMI

After you establish the structural framework described in Chapter 1 and begin conceptualizing the client's problems as described in Chapter 2, you use the three sets of core strategies to address the client's concerns. We begin with the first of these, the change-oriented strategies drawn from behavioral science, especially from the cognitive-behavioral tradition. This chapter tells you how to use change strategies when (1) clients are prone to emotion dysregulation, (2) they have multiple serious, chronic problems and treatment failures, and (3) all of the above occur not only in the client's life but also in the therapy relationship. Typically, you must work simultaneously on many serious problems. For this reason, DBT's target hierarchy and the client's case formulation provide guidelines about *what* to work on and how to allocate your time strategically. What's required is that you treat the highest priority target sufficiently but this need not take up the entire session; most often multiple targets can be addressed within a single session. To work efficiently, you focus attention on the controlling variables that are common across target behaviors and weave change strategies together to address these common processes. In particular, change strategies directly target the client's emotion dysregulation. The therapist often must rapidly assess and improvise to fit the basic change strategies to the moment, giving sessions a sense of movement, speed, and flow. This chapter illustrates how the use of change oriented strategies can be creative, flexible, and precise.

DBT asks the therapist to approach therapy sessions as a jazz musician approaches his or her sessions. Mastery of basics allows improvisation that is both disciplined and free. Just as this requires that the musician over-learn the basics of his or her instrument, the movement, speed, and flow one needs in DBT comes from overlearning the tools of behavior therapy. As described in Chapter 2, the tools you use to determine the controlling variables for problem behaviors are behavioral principles and behavioral assessment. The tools you use to help the client make desired changes are strategies such as self-monitoring, behavioral analysis and solution analysis, didactic and orienting strategies, and procedures such as skills training, exposure, contingency management, and cognitive restructuring (O'Donohue & Fisher, 2009). Table 3.1 lists standard CBT interventions along with the corresponding techniques used within a DBT framework.

As mentioned in Chapter 1, behavioral expertise is required in DBT and this single chapter can't communicate all you need to know. Readers who have not had an opportunity to study behavior therapy should see Wright, Basco, and Thase (2006); Anthony and Barlow (2010); and O'Donohue & Fisher (2006). This chapter briefly describes the standard CBT techniques listed in Table 3.1 before discussing how each is modified when used in a DBT framework.

TABLE 3.1. **Standard CBT Techniques and Corresponding Modifications Made in DBT**

Standard CBT strategies	DBT strategies
Orienting	Micro-orienting
Didactic	Psychoeducation on behavioral principles
Commitment	DBT commitment strategies
Self-monitoring	DBT diary card
Behavioral analysis/functional analysis	Chain analysis
Insight	Biosocial theory and highlighting
Solution analyses	Troubleshooting and generalization
Skills training procedures	DBT skills
Exposure procedures	DBT as exposure
Contingency management procedures	Natural contingencies of the therapeutic relationship; 24-hour rule; four-miss rule
Cognitive modification procedures	Dialectical persuasion, logic, wise mind

ORIENTING AND MICRO-ORIENTING

Most CBT protocols typically begin by orienting the client to the rationale for proposed treatment interventions and by providing straightforward instructions about how to best participate in therapy tasks. Each intervention is vividly linked to the client's ultimate goals so that the client is well oriented about what is proposed, why it is proposed, and how to do it. In DBT you not only orient at the beginning of treatment but also provide what could be called *"micro*-orienting." Because change interventions themselves can be experienced as invalidating, they will evoke emotion dysregulation that may disrupt collaborative work on therapy tasks. Consequently, you must frequently explain why a particular treatment task is necessary to reach the client's goals and, further, you will need to instruct the client specifically on how to do the therapy task despite or in the face of emotion dysregulation.

For example, a client and therapist are assessing what led to the occurrence of a particular instance of target behavior that week. When the therapist asks for details, the client suddenly curls into her chair, head down and mute. This behavior signals emotion dysregulation. In order for assessment of the target behavior to continue, the client needs to be helped to re-regulate her emotion as well as oriented to the original task. This micro-orienting might look like the following:

THERAPIST: Susie, something just happened and you have curled up and become silent. My guess is you've had a huge wave of emotion— maybe fear? Maybe shame?

SUSIE: (*Nods, whispers.*) Both.

THERAPIST: (*Hypothesizes that the client is overwhelmed by emotion and therefore continues in gentle but matter-of-fact manner. In case others have failed to respond to less dramatic expressions of distress and thereby inadvertently shaped the client into an extreme communication style, the therapist attempts to provide a clear, contingent, helpful response with neither an overly solicitous manner or tone nor a punitive or dismissive manner or tone.*) OK, do you know what to do?

SUSIE: (*Shakes her head.*)

THERAPIST: OK, what is needed is to reengage so you can get what you need today. Otherwise, you're likely to feel badly when you leave. Make sense? (*Links rationale for emotion regulation to client goals.*)

SUSIE: (*Lifts her gaze slightly toward the therapist, listening closely.*)

THERAPIST: That probably means you will need to regulate the emotion you are feeling enough to reengage with me. Would you like my help or do you know how to do that on your own—do you know how to take care of yourself and the emotions so that you can come back into the conversation?

If the client in the above example does not know how to downregulate the emotion, the therapist will coach her on specifically what to do. This is shown in the next example, that slowly unfolds over 10 minutes of a later session.

THERAPIST: Susie, were you aware you just changed the topic?

SUSIE: (*Slight smile of fear, slight crumple of body posture.*)

THERAPIST: I think this is one of those places where changing the topic happens automatically, as a way to regulate emotion. I wonder if you feel afraid, maybe? Could that be what's happening?

SUSIE: I guess.

THERAPIST: We could go one of two ways here: we could change the topic or we can continue even though emotion is going up. Remember how we talked about escape conditioning? When a topic gets uncomfortable, sometimes you escape but then you never get the help you need. (*Links intervention to client goals.*) This might be a place to make a deliberate choice to stay with the topic, even if only a little bit longer. To do that, you would throw yourself into the topic again, deliberately talk about what is hard, what you are feeling . . . even right now can you feel how you are holding your breath? See if you can gently take a deep, smooth breath . . . yes . . . again . . . yes, even that is a bit of opposite action to fear (*Uses an emotion regulation skill*). What do you think, a little bit more on this topic?

In another example, client and therapist are doing a chain analysis of a target behavior. In response to a key question, the client gives a very quick "I don't know."

THERAPIST: Sometimes I am not sure what "I don't know" means when you say it that fast. Is it "My mind is blank" or "I'd rather not talk about this" or (*pauses with real curiosity*) . . . something else? What did that "I don't know" mean?

SUSIE: I don't know . . . I mean, I don't know what to say . . .

THERAPIST: Mm hmm, the dilemma is that this is a moment where what you would do next depends on being able to sort out how you feel. So, the thing to do here is to look inside. I asked you, "How did you feel when he said that to you?" and if you slow down for a second, what thoughts do you notice, any body sensations? . . . It's fine to take as much time as you'd like, there's no rush. . . . It could be you need to look without having to have an answer, to search a bit . . .

Such micro-orienting provides the scaffolding to support change-oriented work.

DIDACTIC STRATEGIES

Like other cognitive-behavioral treatments, DBT uses didactic or teaching interventions such as psychoeducation. In DBT you matter-of-factly discuss diagnostic criteria, relevant research, and provide other information that helps the client understand his or her difficulties and the therapy process. In DBT you also directly teach behavioral learning principles, almost as if the client were a graduate student or therapist in training. This is done because the client must not only know how to manage the contingencies that affect his or her own behavior, but also must educate others about how to do so. For example, some clients come to overrely on punishment as a means to regulate their behavior. They have never learned the self-management skills needed to learn, maintain, and generalize new behaviors and to inhibit or extinguish undesirable behaviors. For that reason, the therapist often explicitly teaches principles of behavior change, how to set realistic goals and tolerate limited progress, how to create relapse prevention plans, and, more generally, how to analyze the environment and one's own behavior and to manage the contingencies and stimulus control that can support desired changes (Linehan, 1993a).

Clients must understand such principles of behavior change not only to manage their own behavior but also because treatment providers and others in the client's social network often inadvertently reinforce suicidal behavior and other dysfunctional behavior. For example, one client struggled with chronic suicidal behavior that prompted repeated, lengthy involuntary psychiatric hospitalizations. When the client and outpatient therapist studied the patterns that resulted in hospitalization and patterns that resulted in lengthening the stay after she was admitted, they identified problematic reinforcement contingencies.

Because the client was charming, beautiful, and waiflike, she naturally elicited highly nurturing responses from others. This was a problem. When she acted fragile and passive, problems went unsolved and others moved in to take charge. She then fought their control, ending up in huge power struggles. Her dyscontrol and escalating threats of suicide caused those in her daily life to want her hospitalized. In the hospital, when she acted most vulnerable, the inpatient staff made exceptions and removed demands. Inadvertently, this reinforced her acting fragile and passive. Although done out of kindness and concern, it was an immense disservice. It strengthened the pattern that repeatedly destroyed her outpatient life. When therapy helped her understand how these contingencies increased suicide attempts, she wrote a letter to the inpatient staff. In it, she articulated the problematic pattern of reinforcement that led to extended inpatient stays. She asked that in any future hospitalization, the staff stay somewhat cool and matter-of-fact. In particular, she asked that they refrain from making exceptions for her when she acted fragile or passive and instead asked that they make nurturing contingent on her active engagement with treatment rather than on her passivity or fragility. The client's understanding of reinforcement contingencies was key in changing this pattern that reinforced high-risk behavior.

COMMITMENT STRATEGIES

Explicit, collaborative agreement to work toward mutually determined treatment goals is a hallmark of CBTs and particularly emphasized in DBT. However, getting and keeping such agreement is no small matter. Many clients who come to DBT find it difficult to generate and sustain their motivation to change. Repeated treatment failure has left them defeated and skeptical not only about their own ability to change but also about the therapist's ability to help. Some clients have struggled all their lives to change. They and others have made tremendous efforts, yet have failed. Many clients have learned that therapy offers nothing that produces relief as well or as quickly as intentional self-injury. This makes it hard to give up coping strategies that work, even when the client knows better than you how terribly maladaptive they are. For these reasons, initiating change and sustaining motivation to change will be complicated for many clients.

Therefore, one of the most important tasks of DBT is to help the client become more motivated to make needed changes. Ambivalence about change and lack of motivation to change are expected. They are viewed as problems that the therapy should treat, not ones the client should resolve before being ready to begin therapy. Clients often have a history of coercion and co-optation regarding behavior change; therefore it becomes essential to be exquisitely sensitive to breakdowns in collaboration. You must have the ability to clarify and persist rather than capitulate when met with the client's understandable reluctance or resistance to needed changes. Yet, this must be done in a manner that does not repeat past coercive patterns. The therapist is at times an advocate for new behavior, making compelling and benevolent demands, yet always in the context of a nonjudgmental relationship that supports the client's freedom to choose. This emphasis on building motivation and commitment is shared with a number of CBT approaches (e.g., motivational interviewing and acceptance and commitment therapy).

Consequently, whenever initiating change, especially during initial sessions, DBT emphasizes use of strategies that help clients strengthen their own commitment to change. The following specific commitment strategies are emphasized in DBT as ways to help clients develop and maintain their own commitment to change.

Pros and Cons

Evaluating pros and cons is the meat-and-potatoes strategy that begins work on any target where the client is ambivalent about change. The therapist takes a genuinely balanced stance to help the client consider the reasons for and against change, and the reasons for and against maintaining the status quo. The therapist helps the client explore how the change he or she is contemplating fits with his or her goals and values, particularly exploring any inconsistencies.

Foot-in-the-Door

Foot-in-the-door is when the therapist presents the contemplated change in a vague enough way that anyone would say "Yes." In essence, the therapist frames the change proposition such that the client would say, "Yes, all things being equal, of course I would want that." For example, a client describes how her romantic relationships repeatedly fail, in large part, because she responds to relationship problems by cutting herself. Using foot-in-the-door, the therapist might say, "We could use this therapy to help develop the skills to make and keep better relationships. Would that be of interest to you?"

Door-in-the-Face

Door-in-the-face is the opposite of foot-in-the-door. Here the therapist asks for the moon, the exact or ultimate change needed in the situation without qualification or reservation. For example, using door-in-the-face with the above client, the therapist might say:

> "To have the kind of relationships you want will likely mean completely stopping self-harm. This is an incredibly difficult thing to do, but what I'd propose, is that we go for it, because I can tell how badly you want good relationships. 'Going for it' would mean that for the next year we agree to work together, and as of today you agree to

completely stop self-harm for one year, give it up, and we put all of our energy into finding other ways you can work with these unbearable emotions that come up in your relationships."

Freedom to Choose, Absence of Alternatives

Freedom to choose, absence of alternatives is when the therapist highlights that the client is free to choose whether to make or not to make a change, yet simultaneously highlights highly undesirable consequences of not changing. Continuing the example above, when the client expresses that it is unfair that she must give up cutting, her one effective way to end painful feelings, the therapist might say:

> "Right, one way would be to give up cutting and find new ways to handle this excruciating, out-of-control feeling when you are in a fight with a lover. But I guess another way might be to put your energy into finding a partner who is OK with you going in the hospital a lot . . . who could tolerate or forgive you when you feel hurt and show that hurt by leaving blood on the bathroom floor . . . "

The key here, however, is that the therapist must genuinely be open and respectful of the client's autonomy to choose, without a whiff of judgment or control.

Linking Prior Commitments to Current Commitments

Linking prior commitments to change to current commitments is just as it sounds. The therapist helps the client notice the similarity of past successful changes and highlights that because the client made one change (e.g., successful past commitments to stop smoking or get off heroin) he has the capability to make another change (stop intentional self-injury).

Devil's Advocate

Devil's advocate is when the therapist takes the position of arguing for the status quo, stating the doubts, concerns, or drawbacks of change. This helps the client find his or her own position on why change is important and become active in identifying the barriers and concerns that may block change.

Shaping

Finally, shaping is the gradual strengthening of the client's commitment. The therapist helps the client experience more frequent, intense, or sustained behaviors of wanting, acknowledging and acting in line with the commitment to change.

Commitment strategies such as these are woven into any discussions in which the client's commitment to change could use strengthening and are emphasized whenever work on a new task begins.

SELF-MONITORING: THE DBT DIARY CARD

While self-monitoring is important in many CBTs, it is essential in DBT. Each day the client uses a standard DBT diary card to monitor and record all primary treatment targets. Both sides of the double-sided diary card are shown in Figure 3.1. One side monitors practice of DBT skills. The other side monitors occurrence of other primary targets (suicidal urges and actions, urges and actions to self-harm), associated emotions, and drug use. The client brings the completed diary card to each session and sessions begin with reviewing the diary card together. The therapist and client develop a shared operational definition of target behaviors to be monitored and discuss how changes in these behaviors link to the client's goals. For example, a shared operational definition might be "self-harm is any intentional self-injury that breaks the skin, leaves a mark, or involves ingesting something with the intent to harm." Stopping the intentional self-injury of cutting might link directly to a client's goals because she reports feeling ashamed when others see her scars; she wishes she had less "screwed up ways of coping," and in the long run intentional self-injury increases her risk of death by suicide.

When each target has been clearly defined, then the client self-monitors the frequency, intensity, or other mutually agreed upon aspects of the target. The client–therapist team uses the information on the diary card to guide treatment. For example, the client rates the intensity with which she or he experienced urges to commit suicide, self-harm, or use substances on a scale from 0 (no urges at all) to 5 (the strongest, most intense urges possible). High scores may indicate either an intense or a pervasive occurrence of urges and clients are to rate the most intense or highest urges experienced on that particular day. The same coding scheme is used for physical pain and emotions of sadness, shame, anger, and fear. The client also rates daily skills use, helping both therapist and client note whether the client is trying skills, finding them helpful, and so on. Apparently unimportant behaviors are early warning signals that the therapist and client monitor closely, the seemingly small responses that in fact open the door to problematic behavior. For example, choosing to join coworkers at the bar for happy hour after a stressful workday, while completely reasonable for most people, was for one client the common step toward ending up using cocaine. This client monitored urges to ask if coworkers were going to happy hour, and "urges to ask about happy hour" became a cue to engage her relapse prevention plan. Keeping doors open to use can include things like retaining drug dealers' phone numbers on one's mobile phone or avoiding accepting responsibilities because the client is anticipating the disruption of a relapse. As in other CBTs, you may add other weekly or periodic standardized measures or measures specifically tailored to the individual as needed.

The diary card can save you from many potential problems. First, clients typically have multiple targets, making it impractical to begin a session with questions about every relevant behavior. Even if you could pose a quick check-in question, and the client could answer efficiently with only the information you needed, time would tick away simply due to the number of problems. The diary card lets you see all primary targets at a glance. Second, when crises dominate therapy, it's easy to miss important details. For example, amid a health crisis or interpersonal crisis you might forget to assess suicidal ideation and thereby fail to learn that it has worsened. Here again the diary card saves you by putting the information right before your eyes without you having to remember to ask about it. The diary card can also provide evidence about progress and the act of reviewing the diary card can shape the client's ability to notice problems and progress.

Further, DBT strongly emphasizes anticipating and overcoming the obstacles that will interfere with the client completing the card. Encourage proactive, practical solutions such as selecting a regular place and time to fill out the diary card each day. Regular attention to such solutions may be needed to shape self-monitoring until it is well established. Compliance will be better when you view the diary card as important (rather than as "paperwork"), and you and the client regularly review and use the information. It matters that you consistently ask for and talk about what the client put on the card.

BEHAVIORAL CHAIN ANALYSIS AND INSIGHT STRATEGIES

As detailed in Chapter 2, behavioral chain analysis is used for case formulation and treatment planning. This is an active and ongoing process. A chain analysis is conducted each time the client reports or engages in an instance of a target behavior. Therapist and client analyze the specific instance of the problem behavior to identify the controlling variables, what alternative behavior would have been more functional, and why that more skillful alternative did not happen.

Dialectical Behavior Therapy
Diary Card

Instructions: Circle the days you worked on each skill

Filled out in session? Y N

How often did you fill out this side? ___ Daily ___ 2-3x ___ Once

1. Wise mind	Mon	Tues	Wed	Thurs	Fri	Sat	Sun
2. Observe: just notice (Urge Surfing)	Mon	Tues	Wed	Thurs	Fri	Sat	Sun
3. Describe: put words on	Mon	Tues	Wed	Thurs	Fri	Sat	Sun
4. Participate: enter into the experience	Mon	Tues	Wed	Thurs	Fri	Sat	Sun
5. Nonjudgmental stance	Mon	Tues	Wed	Thurs	Fri	Sat	Sun
6. One-mindfully: in-the-moment	Mon	Tues	Wed	Thurs	Fri	Sat	Sun
7. Effectiveness: focus on what works	Mon	Tues	Wed	Thurs	Fri	Sat	Sun
8. Objective effectiveness: DEAR MAN	Mon	Tues	Wed	Thurs	Fri	Sat	Sun
9. Relationship effectiveness: GIVE	Mon	Tues	Wed	Thurs	Fri	Sat	Sun
10. Self-respect effectiveness: FAST	Mon	Tues	Wed	Thurs	Fri	Sat	Sun
11. Reduce vulnerability: PLEASE	Mon	Tues	Wed	Thurs	Fri	Sat	Sun
12. Build MASTERY	Mon	Tues	Wed	Thurs	Fri	Sat	Sun
13. Build positive experiences	Mon	Tues	Wed	Thurs	Fri	Sat	Sun
14. Opposite-to-emotion action (Alt. Rebellion)	Mon	Tues	Wed	Thurs	Fri	Sat	Sun
15. Distract (Adaptive Denial)	Mon	Tues	Wed	Thurs	Fri	Sat	Sun
16. Self-soothe	Mon	Tues	Wed	Thurs	Fri	Sat	Sun
17. Improve the moment	Mon	Tues	Wed	Thurs	Fri	Sat	Sun
18. Pros and cons	Mon	Tues	Wed	Thurs	Fri	Sat	Sun
19. Radical Acceptance	Mon	Tues	Wed	Thurs	Fri	Sat	Sun
20. Building Structure // Work	Mon	Tues	Wed	Thurs	Fri	Sat	Sun
21. Building Structure // Love	Mon	Tues	Wed	Thurs	Fri	Sat	Sun
22. Building Structure // Time	Mon	Tues	Wed	Thurs	Fri	Sat	Sun
23. Building Structure // Place	Mon	Tues	Wed	Thurs	Fri	Sat	Sun

Urge to use (0–5): _____ Before therapy session: _____ After therapy session: _____

Urge to quit therapy (0–5): _____ Before therapy session: _____ After therapy session: _____

Urge to suicide (0–5): _____ Before therapy session: _____ After therapy session: _____

BRTC Card

Dialectical Behavior Therapy
Diary Card

Initials	ID#	Filled out in session? Y N	How often did you fill out this side? ___ Daily ___ 2-3x ___ Once	Date started

Day & Date	URGES TO...			EMOTIONS					DRUGS				ACTIONS		Joy	Skills	R
	Use	Suicide	S-H	Phys. Pain	Sad Grief	Shame	Anger Irr.	Fear Anx.	Illicit Drugs	ETOH	Prescription	OTC	S-H	Lying	Joy	Skills	R
	0–5	0–5	0–5	0–5	0–5	0–5	0–5	0–5	# Specify	# Specify	# Specify	Specify	Y/N	#	0–5	0–5	✓
Mon																	
Tues																	
Wed																	
Thur																	
Fri																	
Sat																	
Sun																	

Apparently Unimportant Behaviors:

Keeping Doors to Use Open:

*USED SKILLS
0 = Not thought about or used
1 = Thought about, not used, didn't want to
2 = Thought about, not used, wanted to
3 = Tried but couldn't use them
4 = Tried, could do them but they didn't help
5 = Tried, could use them, helped
6 = Didn't try, used them, didn't help
7 = Didn't try, used them, helped

FIGURE 3.1. DBT diary card. Copyright by Marsha M. Linehan. Reprinted by permission.

Reprinted in *Doing Dialectical Behavior Therapy: A Practical Guide* by Kelly Koerner. Permission to photocopy this figure is granted to purchasers of this book for personal use only (see copyright page for details).

Chain analysis is also a major tool to help clients recognize patterns in their behavior (i.e., foster insight). Many clients have developed overly simple explanations for their behavior (e.g., "I'm just lazy," "I'm the kind of person who . . . ") and have absolutely no idea of the controlling variables for their behavior. Similarly, clients often have not had feedback on how they affect others, positively or negatively, and are largely unaware of how their behavior affects others. In DBT, you use chain analysis to teach your client to become actively involved in identifying controlling variables while explicitly teaching a biosocial theory of the etiology and maintenance of emotion dysregulation to destigmatize their difficulties and provide a general idea of what can be done to improve things.

Often, because so many targets need work, the therapist may only have time to briefly highlight patterns, fostering insight as a way to tag something as deserving future attention, or at other times changing its meaning (i.e., stimulus value). The therapist with many higher priority fish to fry might only have time to make a brief comment, such as the following:

"It's interesting—in both of these examples where the other person was being completely unreasonable, the default explanation is that *you* are 'doing it wrong.' Have you ever noticed how often that is the explanation you give for why things don't work out?"

Identifying repeated patterns with the client across different targets can, in some cases, be all that is needed for change. However, the assumption in DBT is that such insight alone is usually not enough to produce change. Instead, emphasis is placed on identifying replacement responses to rehearse and generalize. The client and therapist use solution analysis strategies to generate these alternative replacement responses.

SOLUTION ANALYSES

Solution analysis encourages the client to take an active stance in solving life's problems and strengthens the client's ability to generalize what is learned from therapy to independent use in the client's daily life.

When a client is emotionally regulated, solution analysis is often a straightforward conversation about what the client could do differently. Together you identify desired behaviors or outcomes and then identify the specific steps required to achieve those behaviors or outcomes. You break complex sequences of behavior into doable component parts, that is, using task analysis (as discussed in Chapter 2). You may suggest alternative behaviors, such as specific DBT skills or draw ideas from your own or other's personal experience (e.g., from autobiographies, non-fiction, and films). You can also get ideas for solutions from psychology research (what is normal behavior), treatment research (what works), and psychopathology research (what is likely to interfere with effectiveness).

However, when people are prone to emotion dysregulation or chronic suicidal behavior, the process of solution analysis can require more help from the therapist. It becomes important to teach *how* to solve a problem, especially teaching how to regulate emotion about the problem enough to engage and stay focused during problem solving. In this way, conducting a solution analysis also becomes a vehicle to teach how to regulate emotion while solving complicated problems independently outside of therapy.

Again, in DBT the running hypothesis is that dysfunctional behavior is a *solution*—the client's attempt to solve the problem of emotional pain and discomfort. Whatever the problem behavior, from suicide fantasies, intentional self-injury, back-talking the boss, drinking, or binge eating, it persists because it works: it provides short-term relief. The purpose of solution analysis, therefore, is to identify replacement behaviors that work better for the client—that solve the problem the client has (emotional distress) without the harmful side effects or negative longer term consequences of going for quick relief.

Therapists make a common mistake during solution analysis. We lose track of the fact that a solution must be a solution from the client's perspective, not only from our own. It's easy to misspeak as if stopping the dysfunctional behavior is the end goal. "The goal is to stop cutting." "The goal is to stop binge drinking." But those are not the goals. The goal is for the client to have a life that he or she feels is worth living. For the client, the dysfunctional or target behavior may be a problem, but it is also a solution. The goal is to find a *different* solution, a way to respond to distress that the client views as valuable.

For all of these reasons, you must help a dysregulated and chronically suicidal client with solution analysis more actively than you would a well-regulated client. You must vividly link the new alternative behavior to what matters to the client. When you don't sufficiently micro-orient to rationale, you will lose collaboration. For example, say a client takes much more sleep medication than she should as a way to escape intense distress. She sleeps nearly 24 hours straight, missing work and skills group. From the client's perspective, the overdose worked: it solved the problem of overwhelming emotion. That short-term relief dominates her immediate thinking. Rather than saying, "you need to stop overdosing, let's work on that this session," the DBT therapist would more often frame it as "The problem you solved was emotional distress. What if we worked to find alternative ways to help you? I say this because I know how important it is for you to keep this job and learn as much as you can in skills group." Or, "I think to have the kind of romantic relationships you want . . . " or "Yes, the drawback with overdosing is that I know you feel less respect for yourself when you end up missing work or group." The proposed solution or replacement behavior is linked to the client's goals; it is a means to the client's ends.

When you ask the client to generate solutions and replacement behaviors, you may need to clarify what an adaptive solution would look like as well as directly confront maladaptive solutions. Because the client's solutions are often escape behaviors that produce immediate relief, you frequently must focus on affect tolerance as a solution, as much or more than on solutions that would stop the eliciting events. You may need to systematically help the client predict likely consequences (both short and long term) of various solutions. Avoid solutions that undermine the client's independent realistic problem solving such as suggesting willpower ("just try harder"), overreliance on phone calls to you, and psychiatric hospitalization. Very often you will need to switch back and forth between a focus on solving the client's daily life problems and a focus on assisting in-session emotion regulation. With relentless care and sensitivity, you repeatedly block the client's dysfunctional efforts to escape emotional distress and instead create conditions in which the client shifts toward an active, affective stance toward both life problems and emotion dysregulation, again and again.

Any solution or action plan that is generated must remain feasible even in the face of extreme emotion dysregulation. Troubleshooting potential new solutions becomes essential given clients' problem-solving deficits and severe mood-dependent behaviors (as discussed in Chapter 1). The therapist helps the client anticipate what would prevent the use of the solution and helps identify behaviors necessary for adapting to obstacles along the way.

Therapists typically make errors here. We oversimplify and underestimate how hard it is to use new solutions when emotionally dysregulated. Using new skills to respond to painful rumination may be possible in session with a supportive therapist but nearly impossible after waking from a nightmare, alone, at 3 A.M. Consequently, the emphasis in DBT is to plan for generalization. Use task analysis to reckon with what is possible and needed when highly dysregulated; frequently relate in-session behavior to daily life; provide session tapes for review; and design behavioral rehearsal assignments for completion between sessions.

CASE EXAMPLE: MICHAEL

Here's a clinical example to illustrate the change strategies discussed so far. Michael missed his last skills training group because he overslept. When he and his therapist examined the circumstances, the therapist learned that Michael had struggled with sleep for years, sleeping 14–18 hours a day during periods of high emotional stress. Michael and the therapist agreed to start moving Michael to more balanced sleep both to make sure he did not miss further skills groups and because this pattern greatly interfered with his quality of life. They agreed to begin with a set rise time each morning (Edinger, 2008) and identified that an early morning skills coaching call, initiated by the therapist, would motivate the client. As the vignette begins, the therapist has in mind past chain analyses of Michael's sleep problems as well as intentional self-injury and an overdose, as shown in Figure 3.2. You can see that, looking across targets, dysregulation of shame and self-invalidation seem to be common links. The therapist will therefore be alert to in-session opportunities to work on these common links as an efficient way to treat multiple serious problems.

THERAPIST: How did it go with the sleep stuff? Last time we agreed that a coaching call first thing in the morning might be helpful. How was that for you?

MICHAEL: (*Speaking haltingly.*) Well, I was up, right? We talked.

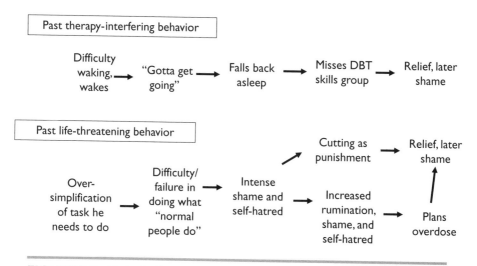

FIGURE 3.2. Michael: Chain analyses of target behaviors in the past.

THERAPIST: Yeah.

MICHAEL: . . . Um. (*Pauses.*)

THERAPIST: Yes, it felt like a stretch to me to do it each morning, but it felt good in that it seemed like you got up, you answered the phone. How'd it go for the rest of your day? (*Communicates briefly about her limits—that her willingness to make "a stretch" is contingent on its being effective.*)

MICHAEL: Well, you know, just knowing you were going to be calling, I'd wake up.

THERAPIST: OK, great.

MICHAEL: So, that was good.

THERAPIST: Good. (*Short silence.*) There's something about the way you're saying it . . . is there something else you want to say about this? (*Gentle laugh.*) Usually you would give me more detail. What's up over there?

MICHAEL: Um . . . well, you know, I . . . well, it's true I was up when you called and I was getting ready to get going with my day, so that was really motivating knowing that you'd be calling. And um, um . . . this is embarrassing. You know, I . . . can we. . . . I think my sleep is actually better, so . . .

THERAPIST: (*Laughs, then in a playful tone.*) What are you avoiding saying over there?

MICHAEL: Well, um, OK, OK. Um . . . when . . . after I got off the phone with you, I was still feeling pretty tired, so I thought I'd lay down and just rest for a little bit and I went to sleep.

THERAPIST: (*Continues in a playful, light tone.*) So you fell back to sleep?

MICHAEL: Yeah.

THERAPIST: You mean your alarm clock went off and you went back to sleep? In essence, me, your trusty alarm clock who went out of my way to call you . . . (*Blocks avoidance behaviors while presenting the cue, trying to minimize feared consequence of overwhelming interpersonal disapproval with playful, light tone.*)

MICHAEL: Yeah. I know, I feel awful about it.

THERAPIST: (*Still light, gentle tone, very present and matter-of-fact.*) I can tell. So, you felt so bad, you weren't even going to tell me, were you?

MICHAEL: Um, I, well . . . I didn't want you to be angry with me, you know. I mean, I feel bad enough as it is.

THERAPIST: Mm hmm.

MICHAEL: You've really been working hard to help me out and I was so surprised when you said that you would try the coaching calls like that . . .

THERAPIST: Yeah.

MICHAEL: . . . And I could tell that you've been frustrated with me all this time because this has been such a huge problem and I can't get things done and so, so you're calling me and like that meant so much to me, and then, you know, I'm a loser, wow.

THERAPIST: So you felt disappointed in yourself . . .

MICHAEL: Yeah.

THERAPIST: . . . And embarrassed to tell me. And it sounds like you're also worried I'm getting frustrated.

MICHAEL: Well, you are. I can tell, you know, I can tell.

THERAPIST: Hmm. Well, actually, I'm not feeling frustrated with you, but I get that you are worried I am. What do you think I'm frustrated with?

MICHAEL: With me. I mean, I'm just not . . . you know, geez, I'm not getting better, and this is a simple thing, you know. People wake up and eat breakfast and they go to work, you know, how many hundreds of millions of people do that every day.

THERAPIST: Mm hmm.

MICHAEL: I've got my therapist calling me, and I'm still back to sleep for 3, 4, 5, 6 hours sometimes.

THERAPIST: Yeah (*Clearly ponders, then speaks slowly.*) . . . it didn't go perfectly. But it did work to get you up. It seems like you're thinking that somehow the whole thing is problematic. I would not say that. I would say that we got part one of the problem solved, which is you got up. Right? It felt motivating and you got up. And then somehow between getting up and getting going, you went back to sleep.

MICHAEL: (*Mumbles.*) But you know, I mean, that's nothing.

THERAPIST: That's what?

MICHAEL: That's just nothing at all.

THERAPIST: What do you mean that's nothing at all?

MICHAEL: I just . . . you know, I just really screwed this up.

THERAPIST: You went back to sleep, yes, you did. Michael, right now, you are feeling guilty and embarrassed and going with the urges of those emotions, kind of going into the whole self-criticism mode. Can you feel that?

MICHAEL: (Nods.)

THERAPIST: To me, if you go with those urges it's going to get us off track, so I'd rather go back and figure this out together. (Blocks self-invalidation, highlights pattern, and micro-orients to the therapy task.) It worked for the first part, you know, like you got up and then how is it that then you went back to sleep? Did that happen every day? (Therapist faces choice of continuing to work on daily life problem or switching to treat what she suspects is beginning of in-session dysregulation similar to what happens across other targets. She opts to see if brief highlighting and her own matter-of-fact tone will help Michael return to the therapy task at hand.)

MICHAEL: Um . . . um . . . well . . . yeah. Every day.

THERAPIST: (Laughs, again a playful, easy manner.) Michael, you've got to do opposite action. Guilt and embarrassment and self-criticism are coming in and they are coming in so strong that they are actually going to get you off solving the problem. And this is probably where it's gone wrong in the past. (Returns to orienting, realizes treating Michael's dysregulation should become the main therapy task.)

MICHAEL: Mm hmm.

THERAPIST: Do you get what I mean?

MICHAEL: That I get so guilty and embarrassed that I don't do anything different.

THERAPIST: Yes, and right now, the action urge you have is to hide, right? Sort of tell me what I want to hear somehow and change the topic . . . ?

MICHAEL: Yes.

THERAPIST: And if you do that, go with the action urge, what's likely to happen with this problem?

MICHAEL: It won't change.

THERAPIST: Right. If you go with the action urge, then you never get the help you need, you never get to actually solving it. (Links Michael's problem behavior of allowing dysregulation to not achieving his goals.)

MICHAEL: Yeah.

THERAPIST: So, what about opposite action right now to the embarrassment or shame? Like I ask you, "Did that happen every day last week, where I called and then you went back to bed?" and you do opposite action to the urge of embarrassment. What would be opposite action? (Offers the solution of using a skill, models, pulls for Michael's active application of a skill to his current situation.)

MICHAEL: You mean, like say it without hiding?

THERAPIST: Yes, answer the question, just very matter-of-fact. Let's try it, "So, did that happen every day?" and you say, "Yes, every day, and I feel so disappointed in myself and worried you'll be frustrated"—just describing without judgment, OK? And shift your body posture to go opposite.

MICHAEL: (*Sits up, puts shoulders back, makes eye contact.*)

THERAPIST: Yes, OK, so, "Did that happen every day?" (*Models and coaches behavioral rehearsal to strengthen skill.*)

MICHAEL: Yes, every day, and I feel so disappointed in myself.

THERAPIST: (*Coaching in quiet voice.*) Yes, see if you can keep the opposite action going, so you can stay in the conversation like that.

MICHAEL: You know . . . I can't take disappointing you more.

THERAPIST: But you're thinking I feel disappointed. Somehow, you're not letting in how I actually feel, which is excited that you woke up. (*Uses contingency clarification.*)

MICHAEL: You're gonna just throw me out of the therapy. I know this is going to happen.

THERAPIST: (*Stays in coaching tone of voice.*) OK, so better here would be just describing, "And I'm having a lot of worry thoughts: I assume you are frustrated; I worry you will kick me out." (*Ticks off thoughts on fingers.*) Try describing thoughts as thoughts, here, OK—still doing opposite action, OK?

MICHAEL: I am having a lot of worry thoughts, and I'm scared that if I don't change faster you will kick me out.

THERAPIST: OK, yes, that's it. Embarrassment and guilt fire, and they usually overwhelm you, and you are doing great here. So, now, really stay with me, OK? The action urge is to only hear what is consistent, what goes right along with the emotion, and I want you to do opposite there, too, which is to really let in, in an open way, what I am saying. Ready? So, what I actually feel is excited because we got the first little inkling. . . . It's been years, right, since you reliably woke up every morning? And you woke each morning this week. (*Changes back to quieter coaching voice.*) OK, so opposite action here, is just to paraphrase, to really get exactly what I said.

MICHAEL: You're excited that I got up every day even though I went back to sleep.

THERAPIST: Right, I view that as the first step. And what I think is that you are not taking seriously how hard this is. You start to get down on yourself and oversimplify it. (*Highlights client's pattern of self-invalidation.*)

This is not an easy problem to solve. You're thinking you're just like all these other people. That is not true. Once anyone gets in this kind of groove or habit of a dysregulated sleeping pattern, it's very hard to change. So, let's just go back and figure this out together. There you were, you woke up. Now, when you woke up, did you have it in your mind that you should stay awake? (*Shifts back to active work on sleep problem, so that in session Michael rehearses the sequence of regulating emotion with opposite action, letting go of self-invalidation and returning to discussing difficult problem, over and over.*)

MICHAEL: Um . . . no.

THERAPIST: OK. I think this is where we missed the boat on our solution last time. I think what we should have tried is a phone call plus finding a "one–two–three" plan of what you're going to do that's going to actually get you momentum. (*Begins task analysis, imagining exactly the steps required in getting out of bed, given Michael's extremely established pattern of disrupted sleep cycles.*) You know what I mean? It's like rolling a big, heavy rock. We rocked it up out of its rut but didn't get it rolling. And what we've got to do is kind of get you all the way up and then rolling with momentum. What would have helped?

MICHAEL: (*Interrupts the therapist.*) But that's just . . . I mean it makes sense that if I'm up, you know, like a normal person would be up and they'd just be up. So, I mean . . .

THERAPIST: Uh-huh, so you're . . . right now you're doing the self-invalidation thing again.

MICHAEL: Well, it's true.

THERAPIST: I know.

MICHAEL: It's true.

THERAPIST: Is that helping you? Is going with that action urge going to help you solve this problem?

MICHAEL: I . . . well . . . the thing is, sometimes things are just true and I think maybe—

THERAPIST: (*Interrupts.*) I'm not disputing that. I'm not disagreeing. Most people do this. I'm not saying that's not true. I'm just saying—is that a particularly helpful thing right this second? Or is opposite action better? You could go back and answer my question, right? What would have helped? There you are, you wake up, we're on the phone, if I had. . . What would have been the one–two–three where, no matter what, you would actually be up, moving through your day? What do we have to do? (*Blocks self-invalidation that she views as avoidance and repeatedly pulls for active problem-solving response.*)

MICHAEL: (*Silence.*) Um, you know, I wish I knew for sure.

THERAPIST: It doesn't have to be for sure. I'm asking for your best guess.

MICHAEL: I . . . you know, what you said, a one–two–three routine sounds like it might be worth a try. So, what am I going to do next?

THERAPIST: Right, what would you need to do . . . if we had a very good routine for you in the morning that would get you going and out that door, what would it be? (*Attempts to "drag out new behavior" from client, active solution generation.*)

MICHAEL: (*Pauses, thinking.*) Um . . . well, you know, if I could eat breakfast, but I'm never hungry when I wake up in the morning. Then I hate eating.

THERAPIST: OK, not breakfast. Keep going.

MICHAEL: Um.

THERAPIST: Just generate as many ideas as you can.

MICHAEL: Well, I don't know . . . put on the TV, put on a morning show or something. Um, I guess . . . like make sure there's a lot of lights on.

THERAPIST: OK.

MICHAEL: TV on. Um, yeah, coffee . . . it's always such a pain to make it, but you know, if I have coffee, I will pretty much stay up if I have coffee.

THERAPIST: Is that right? That's the foolproof one?

MICHAEL: I . . . you know . . . maybe, maybe, maybe.

THERAPIST: Maybe. OK. Do you have an automatic coffeepot?

MICHAEL: No.

THERAPIST: Do you have the twenty bucks it would take to get an automatic coffeepot?

MICHAEL: Um, I . . . I could do that, yeah.

THERAPIST: Could you do that this afternoon? How would it be . . . just imagine this . . . how would it be if you . . . if we agreed again on a time I would call, then the night before you set up your coffeepot. I give you a call, your coffee has brewed, so it's done by the time I call. You get up, you turn on all the lights, you shut the door to your bedroom, and you say to yourself, "You may not go back in there" and you go and fix yourself a cup of coffee.

MICHAEL: (*Quietly.*) You're not leaving me any choice.

THERAPIST: Beg your pardon?

MICHAEL: (*A little more loudly and with a twinkle in his eye.*) You're not leaving me any choice.

THERAPIST: About what?

MICHAEL: Well, about going back to bed.

THERAPIST: (*Catches the client's playful tone, but also checks collaboration.*) I thought we already agreed that was your goal? Are you feeling coerced here?

MICHAEL: No, I know. Yeah, I know. (*Michael and the therapist laugh.*) It's hard!

THERAPIST: It *is* hard. That's my point to you. The easier path is there every morning, you know, stay safe, under the covers, dozing . . . (*Attempts to strengthen commitment by highlighting freedom to choose.*)

MICHAEL: (*Firmly.*) No. I don't want that. You know, I get it.

THERAPIST: It *is* hard. I think you might not be getting how hard, Michael. There's a way where you keep thinking this should be easy, like you should just get up, you shouldn't need any help, just get up. But that's not how it works. It *is* hard. That's why I think I don't feel frustrated. This is a superhard problem to change; it takes repetition to find solutions that will really work. And also there's a whole way that self-invalidation and the action urges of guilt and embarrassment, all of that overwhelms you. . . . You get so dysregulated that you can't move forward on things that matter to you.

MICHAEL: Mm hmm.

THERAPIST: And that's OK. We'll get this. You just did a good piece of work here. (*Senses that self-invalidation is interfering with the client noticing progress in the moment so actively validates and is warm to help strengthen this sequence of effective client behavior.*)

MICHAEL: (*Silence.*) OK.

THERAPIST: Yeah?

MICHAEL: All right. (*Makes good eye contact, is more grounded.*)

THERAPIST: I feel really good about how you just hung in here, too. (*Michael takes a deep breath, relaxes, smiles.*) You used opposite action, you let go a little of self-invalidation, and we got our next idea to try, really nice work. That's the sequence we need. So, now what we should do is troubleshooting. . . . So, let's review: what are you going to do? What's the plan?

MICHAEL: OK, um, yeah, so the coffeemaker, I'll get that today. And OK, I know that many times I've said I'm going to go home and do something, and I don't do it—but I'm going to get it before I go home.

THERAPIST: (*In coaching voice.*) OK, nice opposite action there! Very matter-of-fact, nice.

MICHAEL: When I'm on the way home from this session. I'm going straight to the store.

THERAPIST: OK. Anything you can imagine that would get in the way?

MICHAEL: Um, I don't know. Um, the bus gets into an accident. I don't know.

THERAPIST: (*Laughs.*) How about you get . . . you fall out of the mood. What are you going to do when that happens?

MICHAEL: (*Silence.*) I don't know.

THERAPIST: You *will* fall out of the mood. Let's imagine you all of a sudden are not in the mood anymore.

MICHAEL: Well, I can . . . (*pause*) opposite action.

THERAPIST: Like today?

MICHAEL: Yes.

THERAPIST: OK, think: what will be the emotion?

MICHAEL: I'll feel tired and I'll think, I should be able to do this, this is not a big deal, I shouldn't need a fancy coffeepot—just get up. (*Voice becomes more harsh and unyielding as he speaks.*)

THERAPIST: OK, terrific. Those self-invalidating thoughts will definitely come. That's your cue. Think: What would be opposite action . . . what's the emotion?

MICHAEL: It's kind of like depressed and discouraged, kind of embarrassed, like disgusted.

THERAPIST: So opposite action is . . . ?

MICHAEL: Active, stay active.

THERAPIST: Maybe too, some encouragement, and validation about how hard it is? "It is hard for me to change my sleep. I wish it were different, but it really is terribly difficult." Or even opposite action to disgust—taking a kind, approaching body posture, "I am making a good start on something hard."

As the therapist did the chain and solution analyses of the between-session problem behavior, in-session avoidance behavior began that seemed identical to the exact problem Michael had outside of sessions. Figure 3.3 shows the therapist's brief sketch of the chain analysis of in-session problem behavior and how she intervened.

As shown in this illustration, solution analysis looks like that used in other CBT protocols but may have greater emphasis on blocking avoidance, in-session coaching of regulation, and attention to generalization to

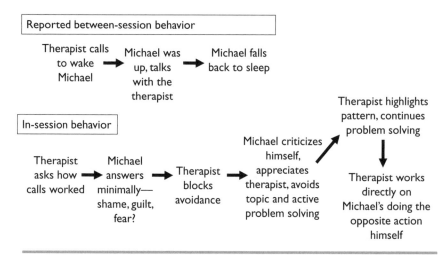

FIGURE 3.3. Michael: Chain analyses of oversleeping and in-session avoidance.

ensure that solutions will actually work in the client's life outside therapy. However, sometimes solution analysis is not enough.

FOUR CBT CHANGE PROCEDURES AS USED IN DBT

One of four factors may interfere significantly enough in client behavior change that more in-depth work is needed before a new solution can be implemented: (1) skills deficits, (2) problematic emotional responding, (3) problematic contingencies, or (4) problematic cognitive processes. Each of these factors links to basic CBT procedures: skills deficits are addressed with skills training procedures; problems with conditioned emotions are addressed with exposure procedures; faulty contingencies are addressed with contingency management procedures; and problems with cognitive processes or content are addressed with cognitive modification procedures. When chain analysis and solution analyses are insufficient in themselves to support new behaviors, one or more of these four basic CBT procedures may be needed.

These four sets of procedures can be infinitely combined, and manualized CBT protocols them for many specific disorders and problems (e.g., Beck, Rush, Shaw, & Emery, 1979; Zinbarg, Craske, & Barlow, 2006; Fairburn, 2008). While you may at times use a full protocol in a step-by-step fashion with DBT clients, most often you will be weaving the principles and procedures in briefer bouts of work, getting as much progress as you can amid crises and work on multiple chronic problems. In the next section, brief definitions of each change procedure are followed by an illustration of how it might be used or given a different emphasis within a DBT framework.

Skills Training

First, the chain analysis may show that the client has a skills deficit, that is, the client does not have the necessary skills in his or her repertoire. Specific skills deficits are targeted in DBT skills training to help with: (1) regulating emotions; (2) tolerating distress; (3) responding skillfully to interpersonal conflict; and (4) observing, describing, and participating without judging, with awareness, and focusing on effectiveness (mindfulness skills). Although clients do most of their learning of DBT skills in skills training classes, the individual therapist also teaches skills, as needed. However, the emphasis for the individual therapist is to strengthen what the client has learned in skills group and generalize skills to the client's daily life problems. The skills trainer gets the skills into the person; you, the individual therapist, pull them out. In the example with Michael, the therapist does this with the emotion regulation skill "opposite action to emotion." This is Linehan's (1993b) shorthand rendition of many evidence-based protocols for anxiety, depression, and anger and expanded to other emotions of shame, guilt, and envy.

As with other CBTs, you instruct the client with easy-to-follow steps and shape the client's responses to more and more closely resemble the desired skilled response. As you and the client discuss the client's life problems, suggest use of DBT skills as solutions. Model and demonstrate skills and help the client rehearse new behavior using imaginal practice or covert rehearsal; brief, impromptu rehearsal (e.g., "he says X, and then what do you say?"); and role play. Informally model use of DBT skills by disclosing examples of how you used the skills yourself. You might also direct the client to other skillful models in the environment (in books, movies magazines, TV) and use stories, metaphors, and analogies. Coach and give detailed, honest feedback that suggests specific refinements so that the skill will work correctly for the client.

Again, behavioral rehearsal is crucial. You'd never consider insight alone to be enough to change your golf swing or paint with oils. Yet we often think that insight alone is somehow enough to change the complicated, highly habitual maladaptive behaviors of regulating emotion. In DBT, practice and overlearning are essential to regulating emotion. Consequently, when the client becomes dysregulated in session, it is a practice opportunity rather than a barrier and a hassle. You move in with direct instruction about how to engage in the therapy task, providing explicit guidance on how to regulate the emotion. Rather than think of somehow getting rid of the dysregulation so you can get to the real stuff with your client, in DBT working with emotion dysregulation *is* the real stuff. Treat it each and every time you get the chance.

The dialogue with Michael offered one example of skills training in the context of in-session dysregulation. Here is another brief one. In this case, the client described the chain of events that ended in bingeing and purging. A key link appeared to be a dysphoric mood and thoughts of "It doesn't matter, nothing matters." As the client recounted the situation, she experienced this same dysphoric mood in session. When the therapist turned the conversation to consider how she might handle the situation differently next time, the client said in a quiet, defeated voice, "What's the point?" The therapist uses this as an opportunity to practice skills.

THERAPIST: What just happened? You just finished telling me about this, and I say, "OK, let's see what we can do about it," and then what happened? What are you feeling?

CLIENT: Nothing's going to help. Why go through all this?

THERAPIST: That's the thought. What's the emotion you're feeling?

CLIENT: (*Silent, while therapist waits.*) . . . I don't know.

THERAPIST: My guess is it's despair and fear, sort of fatigue and overwhelmed, too.

CLIENT: (*Silent.*)

THERAPIST: Listen, this is life-and-death. (*Leans forward, quiet but intense.*) This is what gets you every time, not just with bingeing and purging but also when you want to kill yourself. You've got to find a way to get active here and hang in the conversation so we can figure it out. (*Orients and pulls for active problem solving and also targets a key mechanism tied to suicidal behavior, namely, the sinking sensation/mood that the client labels "Nothing matters!"*) Think for a minute. I say, "Let's do something about this," and you feel what?

CLIENT: It's not worth it, I'm not worth it.

THERAPIST: You look very sad when you say that . . . and then it's like your jaw hardens into resignation . . . yes?

CLIENT: Exactly.

THERAPIST: If you're feeling like this and you're going to try to get yourself not to purge, not to give up, what would it take?

CLIENT: I'd have to feel good about myself, like all of this is worth it.

THERAPIST: All right. What makes it worth it, what can you feel good about?

CLIENT: I don't know.

THERAPIST: Listen, you've got to find something, it has to be genuine, something you really believe. When you get to this point, you've got to be able to find something to feel good about. You know the skill of going to "wise mind," right? Take a deep breath, ask "What can I feel good about?," and listen for the answer, don't make one up, just listen for the answer.

The therapist stayed with the task until the client generated several things about herself that she genuinely valued and this shifted her in-session mood. Then together they thought about how she could do this in her life outside therapy (e.g., what would cue her to remember to focus on things she genuinely values about herself to fight off the despair rather than give in to the mood). Finally, the therapist programmed in gener-alization of the skills by teaching a variety of skilled responses to each situation, varying the training situation, and encouraging practice in all relevant contexts.

Exposure Procedures

Conditioned emotional responses of shame, guilt, unwarranted fears, or other intense or out-of-control emotions often inhibit or disorganize more skillful responding. The person may be "emotion phobic" with devastat-ing patterns of avoidance and escape. In a meaningful way, all of DBT is guided by exposure therapy principles. When formally using exposure procedures, the therapist and client identify the cues that trigger prob-lematic emotional responding as well as escape and avoidance behav-iors. Then the client learns to stay in the presence of the cues without escape and other impulsive actions that function to end contact with the cue (response prevention). Instead of escaping from the cue, the client behaves in new ways that are opposite to the action urge of the condi-tioned emotion (e.g., if the conditioned emotion is fear, an opposite action is to approach). The client gradually exposes herself to more and more difficult cues. Of course it's important that the feared event does not in fact happen (i.e., you don't approach the feared dog and get bitten). This is all done in a manner that increases the individual's sense of control over events and of herself and must last long enough for new learning, habitu-ation, or desensitization to occur.

In Stage 1 DBT, few formal exposure protocols are used but the prin-ciples of exposure are used extensively. When clients are exquisitely sensi-tive, the therapist helps the client titrate exposure to the cues and helps the client to recover and reregulate. For example, in the vignette with Michael, the therapist recognizes his subtle and not-so-subtle avoidance behaviors as she asks how her wake-up calls went. She titrates the cue of disapproval by using a warm, playful manner. She then prevents avoidance by blocking self-criticism while pulling for more adaptive responding in the face of the cue and high emotion. This informal use of exposure requires the therapist to use validation strategically. This is discussed at length in the next chapter on validation.

Contingency Management Procedures

Even otherwise well-trained cognitive-behavioral therapists seldom learn how to use learning principles for contingency management. Somehow, this knowledge and skill set have become passé, and devalued. Yet in DBT, you must know how to use contingency management principles, particularly when helping a client negotiate high-risk suicide crises.

The basic idea is that the consequences of our behavior influence what we learn. A tight, contingent relationship between our responses and their effects in the world influences the probability of what we will do the next time we are in a similar context. Take a simple example. If you walk into a pitch dark, unfamiliar room, there are many things you could do. You could bang around aimlessly; you could yell for help. But the highest probability response in a dark room is to feel around for a light switch. If you find and flip the light switch, yet no light comes on, then you may flip it a time or two more. If nothing happens then you stop flipping the light switch because there is no contingent relationship between flipping the switch and the light coming on. The consequence (no change in light) decreases the chance you will continue to flip the switch. If instead the light came on randomly regardless of your action, then you'd also eventually stop flipping the switch because, again, there is no contingent relationship between your behavior and the light. It is the contingency, the if–then relationship that shapes our responses.

The basic principle holds true in situations that are more complicated. For example, in many service delivery systems, different levels of care are contingent on the severity of behavioral dyscontrol. People only get individual therapy by being completely out of control and clients lose access to individual therapists as soon as they are out of crisis and back in control. The contingencies here favor lack of progress and continued crises. When you do poorly, you get more; when you do better, you get less. A much better system would be to make reinforcement (e.g., for many clients this might be more and more in-depth services) contingent on progress rather than on continuation of maladaptive behavior.

The same principle holds true in subtle interactions. Say, for example, that each time I share with you some personally important fact, you look slightly disinterested. I bare my soul—you check your watch. I try again—your gaze wanders out the window. Presented with that if–then contingency, I adapt and learn that expressions of disinterest are contingent on my self-disclosure. Now, this contingency and the learning it produces may or may not be a good thing. If we are working toward me taking interpersonal risks, like disclosing more in order to develop a sense of trust and intimacy, this contingency is problematic. However, say I use self-disclosure like a squid uses ink; I camouflage my escape when things get tense with a spurt of extremely personal information. Then your withdrawal of interest each time I do this could be aversive enough to help me stop hiding and respond differently. The question must be phrased in terms of how the behavior relates to my goal: does the contingency shape the behavior I want to shape in the direction I want to go?

Similarly, the effect of contingently expressing disinterest may differ across people or even within the same person over time. Expressing disinterest may function as *punishment*, that is, it may suppress my self-disclosure. But if I am exquisitely sensitive so that it is uncomfortable to be seen and known, then your slight withdrawal of attention may actually *reinforce* my self-disclosure—when I share something, you remove the slightly aversive intensity of attention, and I learn I can disclose without being overwhelmed. The way you shape my behavior may change over time. If you are helping me take risks to do what's needed to be close to others and I am ultrasensitive to and inhibited by expressions of disinterest, then you may consciously be careful about how you check the clock near the end of the session early in treatment. But later in therapy, you may just as purposefully not be overly careful, so that I can practice persisting even in the face of normal levels of wandering attention. A final important idea is that of "extinction bursts." If charming, funny self-disclosure is an interpersonal dodge, and the therapist responds contingently by expressing disinterest whenever it functions in this way, there might be an extinction burst. The client may increase telling funny stories, much as one might repeatedly flip a light switch before accepting that it isn't turning on the lights.

Much of this learning based on contingencies between our responses and their effects occurs outside of our awareness. For example, if unknown to an instructor you ask the left side of her classroom to smile and look interested and the right side of the classroom to look disinterested, eventually the instructor will drift to the left without awareness that anything is influencing her behavior. Similarly, this kind of shaping happens in session, too, without our awareness. If each time you ask about a topic that is difficult but important to your client's progress he or she becomes so tangential and monotonous in his or her speech that you become slightly confused and bored, then eventually it becomes less likely you will ask about the difficult topic. The client is shaping you to avoid the topic; each time you drift along with a tangential topic you reinforce the client's avoidance. Therapists are no less vulnerable to learning principles than clients are. In each interaction, you are shaping improvement or not.

Therefore, in DBT, the therapist strives to be aware of the contingencies active in therapy and the therapy relationship so that they are used to the client's best interest. For example, there are two explicitly set contingencies meant to help therapists and clients reinforce active problem solving *before* problem behaviors occur: the 24-hour rule and the four-miss rule.

The 24-Hour Rule

The 24-hour rule sets the following contingency: if the client deliberately self-harms, then the therapist will not increase therapeutic contact during the subsequent 24 hours (although he or she does keep any previously scheduled session). This contingency is meant to strengthen the client's motivation to seek contact when he or she needs help refraining from the old solution of self-harm and replacing it with a new solution. This makes potential reinforcement from increased contact with the therapist contingent on improvement rather than contingent on escalating to problem behavior. The 24-hour rule communicates that things do not have to get extreme before getting needed help. This contingency is also meant to reduce the risk that the therapist will inadvertently reinforce self-harm. If the therapist were to become more warm and solicitous, contingent on intentional self-injury, then it may inadvertently increase the chance of self-harm even if the therapist and client are unaware of this contingency, just as the instructor would unawares drift to the left side of the room.

The Four-Miss Rule

The four-miss rule is similarly meant to help motivate client and therapist to preemptively address attendance problems. If a client misses four consecutive sessions of individual therapy or group skills training, then the client is discharged from the program for the remainder of the contracted treatment period (after which time the client could negotiate reentry into the program). The clarity and non-negotiable nature of this rule motivates the therapist to actively assess and address whatever interferes with attendance. Without mobilizing the therapist in this manner, it can be easy to limp along with sporadic attendance that dooms therapy's effectiveness.

The 24-hour rule and four-miss rule specify arbitrary contingencies: no additional contact for 24 hours after a self-harm incident (why not 12 or 48?), four misses and you're out (why not three, or five?). This arbitrariness is in contrast to perhaps the most important use of contingency management: the naturally occurring contingencies between therapist and client in their relationship.

Natural Contingencies of the Therapeutic Relationship

Natural contingencies are the powerful natural consequences that occur within each therapeutic interaction that are also similar to how things work in nontherapy relationships. Self-involving self-disclosure is one way the DBT therapist uses natural contingencies to benefit the client.

Interactions with the therapist or aspects of the therapy itself (e.g., session frequency or length, payment) may evoke some of the same behaviors that trouble the client in other relationships. For example, the client takes an angry, demanding tone when he makes a request of the therapist that is an imposition on the therapist's time. Others in the client's life are turned off and withdraw from him when he does this to them; his angry tirades inhibit others from giving him feedback; he feels lonely and incapable of keeping good relationships. This is a key place to use self-involving self-disclosure to help the client see the contingency between his behavior and its effects. The therapist might say, "Your voice tone sounds quite angry and demanding as you ask me to do this for you. Were you aware of how your tone comes across? When you ask me in this way, it makes me feel less like doing it. If you asked in a way that showed you realize it may be an imposition, you'd get more of what you want from people."

It is beneficial when the client engages in behaviors with the therapist that are similar to those that cause problems in other relationships because a well-known aspect of reinforcement is that the closer in time and place the behavior is to its consequences, the greater the effect of those consequences. The key is to be aware, from chain analysis and formulation in advance, of what you are trying to strengthen and what you do not want to reinforce. For example, in one client's history, others would not respond to his emotional pain unless he became dramatically upset and made extreme statements such as "I'm going to kill myself if she says that again!" The contingency in therapy should be different: you would want to tune in and respond to distress with plenty of help without it having to escalate. Therefore, warmth, care, and attention should be at a good baseline frequency so that low-level requests and expressions of difficulty regularly produce appropriate help. You would closely monitor the client's current vulnerability factors and antecedents so that when the chain to the pattern is triggered, you can quickly attend to emotional pain but block extreme statements. For example, when this client begins to tell you about an interpersonal conflict similar to those that have led to extreme statements and suicide threats, you might say "I'd really like to help you get things to go the way you want in this situation, so that you do not have to escalate but instead really get what you need." You would stay responsive and warm to the client's appropriate expression, and become cooler when extreme statements are made, even actively blocking them. "When you threaten suicide, it makes us have to assess the risk. To me that takes a lot of time and distracts from what's most important, which is that you are upset by a *real* problem—could you tell me about it without the threats?"

What happens close in time to the incident is more likely to affect the behavior's future probability. Treatment effects will be stronger, therefore, if clients' problem behaviors and improvements occur during the session, where they are closest in time and place to the available reinforcement that the therapist can provide. Nowhere is this more visible than when the therapist and client negotiate solutions to problems in their therapy relationship by explicitly discussing how each person's responses reinforce or fail to reinforce the other's motivation and engagement in therapy.

Some people have objections to contingency management, as if deliberately responding in a contingent way is harmful or deceitful. This objection ignores the fact that we are all responding contingently all the time with everyone anyway. If I am sharing something about myself, you are either responding in a way that makes me more likely to continue to share or less likely to continue to share; this happens whether either of us is aware of the effects or not. As therapists, we want to be as aware as we can be so that we harness our responses to the client's benefit rather than simply responding to alleviate our own discomfort. A good base rate of genuinely noncontingent positive regard is a *prerequisite* to effective use of contingency management. Unless the client experiences you as genuinely invested in his or her best interests, contingency management feels manipulative or coercive.

Cognitive Modification

Effective behavior is sometimes inhibited by faulty beliefs and assumptions. In DBT cognitive modification is based on logical consistency or consistency with one's true or wise-mind beliefs (e.g., "Is this belief what I believe in my wisest moments?") and on effectiveness ("Is this belief useful to meet my goals?"). This emphasis on finding what is valid is due in part to clients' sensitivity to invalidation. Focusing intervention on what is wrong with the client's interpretations, especially through

Socratic questioning, is too evocative and aversive for many. Although the DBT therapist may sometimes challenge problematic beliefs with reason or through hypothesis-testing experiments, the emphasis is on cognitive modification through dialectical persuasion—conversations that create the experience of the contradictions inherent in the client's position. For example, in the last chapter a client described getting immediate relief from emotional pain when she burnt herself with a cigarette; she said it was no big deal. The therapist then asked the client would she burn her little niece's arm to help her feel better, if the child was in great emotional pain? The client replied, "I just wouldn't do it. It's not right." The conversation heightened the client's emotional tension and discomfort of holding a double standard. In dialectical persuasion, the therapist highlights the inconsistencies among the client's own actions, beliefs, and values.

In addition, the therapist helps the client develop guidelines on when to trust and when to suspect her interpretations. For example, the skill "check the facts" distills many basic cognitive modification strategies into a self-help intervention. Further, in DBT, the therapist actively teaches the client to become better able to discern contingencies, clarifying the if–then effects of their behavior in the therapy relationship as well as in the client's other relationships. Clients learn to observe and describe their own thinking style and implicit rules, to notice when their thinking is ineffective, and to confront and challenge problematic thoughts in order to generate a more functional or dialectical sense of truth. The client learns to increasingly rely on wise mind, an intuitive knowing that incorporates rational and emotional responses to be effective. In DBT the principal aim is not to find and change problematic schema but rather to weave cognitive modification informally throughout the treatment, with a strong emphasis on valuing nonrational or intuitive knowing as another means of evaluating besides rationality.

All of the basic change-oriented strategies and procedures discussed in this chapter are combined or modified to effectively work with the client's pervasive emotion dysregulation both in session and between sessions. You often must repeatedly orient, explicitly work on commitment to therapy tasks, and focus on behavioral rehearsal to ensure learning and generalization despite emotional dysregulation. You target the links in the chain of causation that are common across problems and situations; you do this by using highlighting, solution analysis, and each of the four change procedures (skills training, exposure, contingency management, and cognitive modification). In each interaction, the client and therapist remedy skills deficits and work to change problematic emotions, contingencies, and cognitions that interfere with skillful responses already in the client's repertoire.

Yet change interventions can be experienced as highly invalidating. The therapist's attempts to help can feel critical and can seem to confirm that the client has not tried hard enough—just as others have always said. Clients with histories of pervasive invalidation can be exquisitely sensitive. For this reason, active, disciplined, and precise validation of what is "right" or "correct" about the client's current responses is required to motivate emotion regulation and thereby create conditions for other change. The next chapter describes validation strategies, the acceptance-oriented core strategies used in DBT.

FOUR

Validation Principles and Strategies

DBT defines validation as empathy plus the communication that the client's perspective is valid in some way. With empathy, you accurately understand the world from the client's perspective. With validation, you actively communicate that the client's perspective makes sense. To validate you must have empathy so you understand the other person's unique, nuanced perspective. But validation further requires that you seek out and confirm that a response is valid. You substantiate how the client's emotion, thought, or action is completely understandable because it is relevant, meaningful, justifiable, correct, or effective. Were the client to ask, "Can this be true?" empathy would be understanding the "this" and validation would be communicating "yes." Validation is the second set of core strategies in DBT. Validation comes from the client-centered tradition (Linehan, 1997b; see also the excellent book *Empathy Reconsidered* [Bohart & Greenberg, 1997]).

It's tempting to view the change strategies in the last chapter as the main engine of therapy, the most important part of the help you offer, as if behavior therapy were a crowbar that needs a counterweight of validation to pry the client toward change. But these views are wrong-headed and simplistic. They miss the powerful change that validation, *in itself,* produces. These views also mislead the therapist into thinking that validation is so naturally part of who we are as therapists that no particular training or practice is required to provide it. In fact, active, disciplined, precise validation is required to motivate emotion regulation and thereby create conditions for other change. When clients come from a history of pervasive invalidation and are currently emotionally vulnerable, providing validation is a lot harder than you'd think.

UNDERSTANDING INVALIDATION'S ROLE IN EMOTION DYSREGULATION

Case Example: Mia

Mia came to therapy to get help with problems at work, but things had gone too far to save her job. When she was subsequently fired, her therapist suspended her usual therapy fee, agreeing that Mia could carry a balance to be paid when she was again employed. Now, Mia is interviewing for a new job. She comes to session and tells the therapist about an interview with a company she'd be thrilled to work for—but the interviewer was impossibly rude and asked her several leading questions to "make her complain about her former employer." The therapist asks what she thinks are innocuous questions to assess the situation and to learn what Mia wants to do next but she does not validate that the interviewer was impossibly rude. Mia repeats the interviewer's questions with a dramatic, cross-examining voice tone, and goes on to say she has already drafted the "thank you for the interview" email, listing each inappropriate thing he said. The therapist thinks Mia is misinterpreting normative ambiguity and voice tone as the therapist has seen happen in therapy. She wants to help Mia tolerate these unavoidable aspects of interviewing. So she says, "Well, I can see that the tone of voice might have been difficult but the questions themselves are common to any job interview." Mia flames into fury. "If you want me to pay the balance I owe you, I will, just say so!" "Whoa!" says the therapist, in a very gentle tone, "No, you are misreading me, I know this interview was super important to you" and then the therapist, anxious to avoid further antagonizing Mia, yet irritated herself, slips into a slightly sing-song voice tone as she tries to mask her own emotional reaction. "Listen, neither the interviewer nor I are trying to trick you . . . but I know these kinds of situations are really confusing for you." Mia experiences this as condescending and humiliating but what flashes across her face is scorn. The therapist is quiet for a moment, trying to regroup and get her bearings in the conversation, which then prompts Mia's wave of panic as she tearfully anticipates the therapist abandoning her and failing to get the help she needs.

For the therapist, validation and even empathy can be difficult in this situation. If we saw the bubble over the therapist's head it might say: "I've believed in you enough to let you owe me money and you attack my motivations?! I've been working my butt off for you." The thought bubble might also say, "If she sends that email, she's heading into a suicidal crisis . . . let me out of here." But Mia has good reason to suspect others' intentions. Repeated lies, public humiliations, and emotional coercion were the norm in her family, grinding her to a suspiciousness verging on paranoia. She is understandably sensitive and likely to misread situations as setups where she will be tricked and harmed. Knowing Mia's history and sensitivity, the therapist gently offers careful feedback, but even sensitive phrasing feels like stomping and torturing to Mia. When treading through such old, overused patterns to clarify misperceptions, the opportunity for therapist missteps is high.

Mia's responses, however, are not just misperceptions that make sense in light of past invalidation; they occur because she is being invalidated, *now*, by her therapist, in this *current* interaction. The therapist's first move is to check whether Mia is misreading the situation, that is, to find what is mistaken or invalid about Mia's responses. This triggers for Mia a rush of responses that could be expressed as, "No one believes me, no one will protect me, I have to protect myself or things like this will keep happening." The emotional quality of her communication intensifies. As the therapist persists, tense and walking-on-eggshells about Mia's emotionality, Mia feels the therapist keeps missing her message about how disturbing this interviewer was. She begins to wonder *why* the therapist doesn't get it, reading correctly that the therapist is tense, but then mistakenly guessing the tension is because the therapist needs her to take the job in order to pay the outstanding therapy bill. When the therapist comments that "these kinds of situations are confusing for you," she again implies that Mia is misreading the situation. To Mia this feels like a humiliating pronouncement. When the therapist gently reminds Mia that she knows how important the job is to Mia, it triggers a dialectical shift to self-invalidation and intense self-contempt: "I'm so stupid, I overreact to everything. Everyone else can keep a job what's wrong with me?!" The look of scorn the therapist saw on Mia's face was self-directed. Then amid all of this, Mia feels the therapist withdraw. The therapist *needs* to withdraw, and does so in order to regulate herself so she can help Mia. The therapist's withdrawal when Mia needs her, however, further amplifies Mia's distress: if she is really as out of control as she feels, then why doesn't the therapist help? Can't she see how bad things are? Mia feels trapped in a nightmare as nothing she does works and the safety of at least having her therapist on her side slips away. As emotional intensity escalates, so does the probability of extreme behavior. The risk is high that the session will go downhill and Mia will leave in worse shape than she came in. This is a typical scenario and can be incredibly demoralizing to both therapists and clients.

The Normative Effects of Invalidation

In the heat of the interaction, it would be hard for any therapist to see what is valid and normative about Mia's increasingly emotional communication and especially difficult to see that it is the therapist's own responses that make things worse. When Mia's initial emotion fires and is followed by the therapist's invalidation (questioning Mia's "read" of the situation), Mia's experience and expression of emotion escalates. *As it would for each of us.* It is a normal psychological process for invalidation to produce increased arousal and the sense of being out of control (Shenk & Fruzzetti, 2011). We have all had a time when we found ourselves more intensely experiencing and expressing emotion after someone doubted our read of a situation. If we are doubted long enough and thoroughly enough about something with high stakes, our emotional experience and expression become extremely intense. We fail to process new information and make intense efforts to regain control. This is *normative.* In the vignette, the therapist fails to reckon with the *normative* response that her invalidation of Mia will produce: emotional arousal.

In the face of such invalidation, depending on our learning history and temperament, we may habitually escalate our emotional expression or we may make automatic or intentional efforts to downregulate our emotion. When emotion is intense but not overwhelming we might interrupt ourselves, blunt, postpone, numb, mask, avoid, withdraw, or selectively focus our attention. We may react to our own responses with scorn, fear, or shame (i.e., have secondary emotions). Those of us with better emotion regulation skills might have very intense emotional experiences but we have the ability to modulate our expression to fit the social circumstance. For instance, Mia's therapist deliberately shifts to a more relaxed body posture and slows her breathing as she notices the beginning of her own dysregulation.

When the stakes are high (as in Mia's example above) and others fail to respond to our emotional communication, we can each be pushed to the point of dysregulation, where we literally or metaphorically have screamed, "You don't understand!" Obviously, not all of us resort to intentional self-injury to solve the problem of dysregulation, but the basic psychological processes are the same for client and therapist. Invalidation sets off heightened emotion, narrowing our perception, thinking, and action urges, focusing us to deal with the threat. The only thing that matters is getting our message across.

For our clients, dysregulated experience and expression may become a habitual, lightning-fast response that in turn rapidly triggers tangled interpersonal patterns. The process may happen so quickly and in such unexpected contexts that as therapists we miss this transition from a cue (e.g., our inadvertent invalidation) to intense emotion. We suddenly find our client in an inexplicably dysregulated state. Everything becomes complicated. Therapy feels like a field of landmines, for both parties.

What is difficult to tolerate, for client and therapist, is that invalidation is necessary—the therapist *must* communicate what is ineffective and does not make sense about Mia's responding. Without the therapist's corrective feedback (e.g., about how to best interpret and respond to an interviewer's behavior), Mia will continue to lose job after job; uncorrected, her misinterpretation of the therapist's motives will corrode her trust in the therapist. Her emotion *is* too strong, both normatively and also practically: it will derail work the two must do to prevent her from precipitously emailing the interviewer. It is not viable to drop the topic. Nor does it help to agree with what's invalid (e.g., "The interviewer sounds like a total jerk, it's outrageous that someone would speak to you that way!"). The therapist must invalidate (or at least avoid validating) emotional responses when they are out of proportion or based on mistaken interpretations.

Helping clients change often requires actively and repeatedly invalidating responses that are incompatible with achieving the client's long-term goals. Yet it is normative for repeated invalidation to produce emotional arousal and eventually dysregulation that interferes with learning and flexible responding. When clients are exquisitely sensitive, how can we best promote change and new learning?

Using validation as you might throw an angry dog a bone won't work in these situations. (Just remember the last time you mouthed a "yes, dear, that must've been hard when I did that" to a loved one who was furious with you.) What's needed is more complex. The therapist must simultaneously align with the client's goals and remain open to what's valid about the client's response, without reinforcing dysfunctional behavior, without evoking such emotional reactivity that the therapeutic task is derailed, and without dropping a focus on needed change. For example, with Mia, the therapist needs to stay open to the possibility that the interviewer's tone was indeed nasty; she might need to validate the extreme emotional experience (the anger fires up so intensely because Mia may be blocked from an incredibly important goal) without validating problematic emotional expression (retaliating by sending the email is not in her best interest).

THE EFFECTS OF ACCURATE, PRECISE VALIDATION

Validation in itself reduces physiological arousal. In other words, validation directly down-regulates emotion (Shenk & Fruzzetti, 2011). Validation in itself also cues adaptive responding that regulates emotion. When you validate, accurately, with precision, you not only reduce arousal but also trigger competing responses. Strongly worded and emotionally evocative validation prompts new, more adaptive emotions to fire, which by definition means that the client's whole system reorganizes. Just as a great writer's word choice evokes emotion, so can the therapist's.

Let's say this way of thinking had guided the therapist when Mia relayed how incredibly rude the interviewer was. The therapist might instead have said, genuinely and with intensity, "How frustrating!! You were so looking forward to this interview, you must be *so* disappointed." How would Mia respond?

MIA: I am! And I'm furious! I had researched everything about the company; I talked for hours with a friend about how to handle the gaps in my work history. Then this jerk ruins it all!

THERAPIST: Oh, Mia, I'm so sorry. I know you put in so much effort to prepare, and were really looking forward to it.

MIA: Yes . . . (*Tears come to her eyes as she realizes how much she had riding on this interview.*) I'm just not going to get chances like these, this is a once-in-a-lifetime thing.

THERAPIST: Yes, this is such a unique opportunity. . . .

MIA: (*Tears welling.*)

THERAPIST: It really hurts . . . um hmm.

The therapist slows down her pacing to promote Mia's full expression of the primary adaptive emotion of disappointment. Mia, crying, takes a deeper breath, and sighs. The therapist also takes a deep breath and sighs, taking the moment to appreciate how hard Mia has been working toward this interview and the extent of emotion she herself would feel if a perfect opportunity were taken away. From this fuller appreciation, she begins to frame change interventions that can be sensitive to the hair-trigger of Mia's emotions, or of anyone's emotions with such a huge potential threat on the scene.

The therapist might then continue:

THERAPIST: You know, right now I feel like there's been an explosion and all the alarms are going off and you're right in the middle of it. Even while you're feeling devastated and crying, you also have your guns drawn ready to shoot the first thing that moves. Am I reading you right? The threat here is so big, you're on full alert, full attack mode?

MIA: (*Nods.*) Exactly! (*Raises her fingers as if pointing guns at the therapist.*)

THERAPIST: Exactly. And I want to say, "Don't shoot my head off! I'm friendly!" (*Puts her hands up.*) Before I say another word, I want to say: "Listen, don't shoot—OK?" (*Turns earnest and intense.*) I know how bad you want this, how hard you worked, how much this means, OK? . . . (*Pauses, holding Mia's gaze.*)

MIA: (*Cries but also smiles and relaxes a little.*)

THERAPIST: Can I put my hands down? Before we go on the warpath, I have an idea . . . OK? You with me?

When the therapist validates, he or she can do so in ways that trigger and reinforce adaptive alternative responses in the very situation where they have been absent yet so needed. At a given moment, multiple emotions may be firing, some at full strength, some weaker. When the therapist directs the client's attention and triggers an adaptive emotion with a validating comment then, by definition, the client's perception, sensing, remembering, and action urges of that emotion also are cued. In other words, validation can cue the full coherent response that comprises the adaptive emotion. By doing so, more flexible, adaptive responding may become immediately possible. In the revised vignette above, validation is guided by the intent to both downregulate arousal and cue adaptive emotions. In combination, they make a productive conversation possible with Mia in an emotional but not dysregulated state.

Precise validation can be incredibly powerful, yet incredibly difficult to do when most needed. Therefore in this chapter I'll break things down. First, I'll describe in general what to validate when people are prone to emotion dysregulation. Then, I'll give you four guidelines for using validation strategies: (1) search for the valid; (2) "know thy client"; (3) validate the valid and invalidate the invalid; and (4) validate at the highest possible level. Then with these shared basic concepts in mind, we'll look at how to use validation to strengthen emotion regulation, concluding with an extended clinical example to show how validation and change strategies are combined.

WHAT TO VALIDATE

When a Client Is Emotionally Dysregulated

In nearly all situations and with nearly all clients, you can assume it will be welcome if you validate that the client's problems are important (*problem importance*), that a task is difficult (*task difficulty*), that *emotional pain* or a *sense of being out of control* is justifiable, and that there is *wisdom in the client's ultimate goals*, even if not in the particular means he or she is currently using.

It is essential to validate clients' *location perspective*, that is, their views about where they are, their current views about life problems, and beliefs about how changes can or should be made. Unless the client believes that the therapist truly understands the dilemma (e.g., exactly how painful, difficult to change, or important a problem is) he or she will not trust that the therapist's solutions are appropriate or adequate. Collaboration will be limited and so too the therapist's ability to help the client change.

Say you are away at a conference and you get an emergency page. You phone the number and an emergency room nurse answers and tells you someone you love dearly has been terribly hurt and you must sign the release before needed medical attention can take place. You begin to get directions to the hospital. The nurse tells you to "go to the highway and then head south until you come to . . . " But you tuned her out as soon as she said "south"—you think the conference location is such that you actually need to catch the freeway and head *north*. You try to communicate this. She says, "Oh, no, just catch it south and then . . . " You have a rising sense of panic; she isn't listening! She doesn't know where you are. She *must* understand where you are before she can help you get where you need to go. You intensify your emotional expression—the stakes are tremendous.

It is often like this for our clients. They have a sense of where they are; we then begin to provide directions that feel as if we don't know where they are. We persist. It is infuriating and terrifying for our clients. It matters who has the client's correct location and where that location is relative to where the client wants to go. If that emergency room nurse is right, she needs to win the argument—she will have to calm you by clearly showing you she knows exactly where you are. But if you are right, the nurse must be open to your influence. Often a rift in collaboration comes from exactly this type of disagreement about the client's location relative to their goals, thus it is essential to validate and get consensus on location.

When a Client's Response Is Both Valid and Invalid at the Same Time

You will often need to communicate how the same response is simultaneously valid *and* invalid. The response of self-hatred may be relevant and justifiable (valid), yet at the same time ineffective (invalid) because it is incompatible with the balanced problem solving required to keep oneself from doing the hateful behavior again. Or, for example, say you've forgotten some fact that's important to a client without being aware you have done so. As the conversation continues, the client becomes overly cheery and stops saying anything of substance about the topic. When you wonder aloud about the change in mood and depth of the conversation, the client airily dismisses your concern. The client's response may be valid in terms of past learning history (e.g., if her cultural background prohibits drawing attention to another's failings or directly expressing irritation about them) or current circumstances (if your tone is even slightly defensive or accusatory and it's logical to infer you won't be open to the feedback). But simultaneously, her response is invalid if it fails to prompt you to correct your behavior when you need the fact to help her.

When It's Hard to See Anything Valid

When it is hard to see what's valid about a response, first look for how it might be relevant and meaningful to the context. In the context of psychotherapy, curiosity about whether my therapist has kids is relevant if I am assessing if she will understand my struggles as a parent (chitchat about the Mariners' new shortstop is not). Sometimes therapists are trained to be suspicious of such curiosity. To validate means to attend to how such questions are relevant, not pathological. Second, see if the response is well grounded or justifiable in some way. Look for the *facts, logical inference, or generally accepted authority* that makes the response sensible. It is logical for a client to infer that I am irritated with him if I greet him less warmly in the waiting area after he has left me a phone message full of personal attacks and criticism. Third, search for how a response is *an effective means* to obtain some immediate end. Even patently invalid behavior may be valid in terms of being immediately effective. Cutting one's arms in response to overwhelming emotional distress makes sense, given that it often produces relief from unbearable emotions: it is an effective emotion regulation strategy. Of course, a response can be valid in more than one way. When a client says she hates herself, hatred is both relevant and justifiable if the person violated her own important values (e.g., had deliberately harmed another person out of anger). Ultimately, every response is valid in terms of historically making sense—all factors needed for the behavior to develop have occurred: therefore, how could the behavior be other than it is?

Other Validation Targets

In any given situation, you can validate emotional, behavioral, or cognitive responses as well as the client's ultimate ability to attain goals. For adaptive emotion regulation, one must experience and express primary emotions. Validation is required to develop this ability. Therefore, read the client's emotions, directly validate primary emotions (e.g., "feeling sad makes sense"), and encourage emotional expression. Observe and label clients' emotions (e.g., "Your eyes look teary; I wonder if you feel sad right now"). This helps to teach client these skills.

To validate behavioral responses, observe and label behaviors. For example, observe when demands are self-imposed; standards for acceptable behavior are unrealistic; and guilt, self-berating, or other punishment strategies are used (identify the "should"). Counter the "should" (i.e., communicate that all behavior is understandable in principle). Accept the "should" (i.e., respond to the client's behavior nonjudgmentally and discover whether there is truth to the "should" when phrased as "should in order to").

To validate cognitive responses, elicit and reflect thoughts and assumptions, find the "kernel of truth" in the client's cognitions, acknowledge the client's intuitive ability to know what is wise or correct (wise mind), and respect the client's values.

To validate the person's ability to attain desired goals, assume the best, encourage, focus on strengths, contradict/modulate external criticism, and be realistic in assessment of capabilities. (I've always liked Linehan's [1993a] use of "cheerleading" for this type of validation. Whether your team is up by 14 or losing badly in the last minutes, on a muddy field—your response as a cheerleader is the same. Right there on the sideline until the whistle blows, there on the bus home, there at the next practice.)

The above guidelines on what to validate are summarized in Table 4.1. Now, with these concepts in mind, let's break the complex use of validation strategies into four component steps.

TABLE 4.1. What to Validate

- The client's primary emotional responses and expressions
- The client's behaviors: observe and label
- The client's cognitions: reflect his or her thoughts, assumptions, and values
- The client's ability to attain his or her ultimate goals

When a client is dysregulated, validate:
- The problem's importance
- The task's difficulty
- The client's emotional pain
- The client's reasons for feeling out of control
- Wisdom in the client's ultimate goals (if not the means selected)
- The client's location perspective

When it's hard to see what to validate, validate:
- Past learning history
- Whatever is justifiable in terms of facts, logical inferences, or accepted authority
- Whatever is an appropriate or effective means to an end

HOW TO VALIDATE

Search for the Valid

Actively search for what is valid, and assume that there always is *something* valid. You don't make the client's response valid. You *find* what is valid. "The therapist observes, experiences and affirms but does not create validity. That which is valid pre-exists the therapeutic action" (Linehan, 1997b, p. 356).

Know Thy Client (and the Psychopathology and Normal Psychology Literatures)

Be aware of what is valid and invalid for the specific client. This is where a thorough grounding in psychological science to understand what is normative and how psychopathology develops and is maintained becomes a true asset for therapists. Remember your case formulation, especially, the emotion sequences that are habitual for this client—what are likely primary emotions and secondary emotions for this particular client? Constantly be aware of the client's current emotional arousal and how it affects the ability to process new information, then balance change and validation accordingly.

Validate the Valid; Invalidate the Invalid

Be precise about what you are validating. For example, Bettina is thinking of moving in with the archetypal Bad Boy she met this weekend after he charmed her at the dance club (the fourth Bad Boy in the last 3 months). She asks that all of today's session focus on how to hang on to this relationship. As has happened before, Bettina cancelled plans with friends and blew off important obligations in case the new boy called, and she had no energy to further her job search. From past experience, this situation is a looming disaster in Bettina's parents' view. What is invalid may jump out at you and you may come to ignore or trivialize her feelings of love and the intense desire she has to make this relationship work. But dismissiveness invalidates both the valid and invalid aspects of the request.

Instead, validate the valid (perhaps identify the wisdom of the ultimate goal of romantic love or of the specific qualities she is attracted by) while invalidating the invalid (e.g., by insisting that the session agenda include an adequate plan to proactively address the life crises). To invalidate the invalid, be descriptive and nonjudgmental, articulating how the response does not make sense or does not work. For example, Bettina's therapist might say:

"I agree—one of our most important goals is helping you have intense loving relationships that really work for you, and one aspect of that is that when a new love starts you lose all motivation to work on things that give you self-respect. This increases self-hatred; then you feel more needy and put incredible pressure on the lover to make you feel good about yourself. If we're not smart about our session time today, things could go downhill in a hurry. "

When you can genuinely, with empathy, describe both what is valid and what is invalid, you don't need to walk on eggshells. You can go "where angels fear to tread," freed up to tell it like it is without alienating your client.

Validate at the Highest Possible Level; Actions Speak Louder Than Words

Linehan (1997b) distinguishes six levels of validation (described below); Level 6 is the highest. At each level, do not rely solely on explicit verbal validation: nonverbal expressions are both required and often more powerful. In other words, if you were trapped at a 4th-floor window of a burning building, and a firefighter showed interest, accurately reflected your distress, and genuinely communicated how it made sense, it would still be insufficient! What you need is for him to grab your arm and get you to safety. Functional validation—responding to the client's experience as valid, and therefore compelling—is essential. Verbal validation alone, when functional validation is required, is an error often made by therapists.

Level I: Listen with Complete Awareness, Be Awake

Listen and observe in an unbiased manner, and communicate that the client's responses are valid by listening without prejudging. So, for example, the therapist hears Bettina's request to talk about a love interest as if it were completely new, without construing it solely in terms of a pathological recurrent pattern.

Level 2: Accurately Reflect the Client's Communication

Communicate understanding by repeating or rephrasing, using words close to the client's own without added interpretation. Remain nonjudgmental, that is, not focused on improvement or encouragement or evaluating effectiveness or merit, but instead on the simple "is-ness." "This is how it is for you right now."

Level 3: Articulate Nonverbalized Emotions, Thoughts, or Behavior Patterns

Perceptively understand what is not stated but meant without the client having to explain things. Clients with a pervasive history of invalidation are so sensitized that often they disclose a tiny bit but feel they have told you everything; or so habitually mask or control expression that you need to intuit the rest from small signals. Greenberg (2002) reprinted a quote from Truax and Carkhuff (1967) that captures what is aspired to in these first three levels of validation. The validating therapist:

> (U)nerringly responds to the client's full range of feelings in their exact intensity. Without hesitation, the therapist recognizes each emotional nuance and communicates an understanding of every deepest feeling. The therapist is completely attuned to the client's shifting emotional content, senses each of the client's feelings, and reflects them in words and voice. With sensitive accuracy, the therapist expands the client's hints into full-scale (though tentative) elaboration of feeling or experience. (Greenberg, 2002, p. 78)

Level 4: Describe How the Client's Behavior Makes Sense in Terms of Past Learning History or Biology

Identify the probable factors that caused the client's response. For example, to a client who constantly seeks reassurance that therapy "is going okay," the therapist might validate by saying, "given the unpredictability of your parents, it makes sense to have the feeling of waiting for the other shoe to drop and seek reassurance."

Level 5: Actively Search for the Ways That the Client's Behavior Makes Sense in the Current Circumstances, and Communicate This

Find the ways a response is currently valid, whenever possible, and remember not to rely only on verbal validation. For example, say you were walking to a movie theater with a friend who'd been raped in an alley, and you proposed that you take a shortcut through an alley so that you wouldn't be late for the movie and your friend said she did not want to because she was afraid. Saying, "Of course you're afraid, you were raped in an alley, how insensitive of me" would be a Level 4 validation. Saying, "Of course you are afraid, alleys are dangerous, let's walk around" would be a Level 5 validation. When you can find a Level 5 validation (and search like a fiend for it), use it rather than a Level 4. Especially here, remember that *you* may in fact be the source of current invalidation. So, for example, with the client seeking reassurance, the therapist might search for ways that he or she is communicating ambivalence or in some other way cuing the client's anxious response, so that seeking reassurance is sensible. Validating in terms of the past (unpredictable parents) when in fact there are aspects in the current situation (therapist ambivalence) prompting the response is experienced as extremely invalidating. ("Yes, yes. I know you are angry with me, but could we discuss how this reminds you also of your family of origin?") Level 5 is like saying, "This response is *not* completely screwed up; here is how it makes sense *now* in the current context." Level 5 is the antithesis of pathologizing. Instead of emphasizing what's wrong, you find what is effective, adaptive and relevant about the response in the current circumstance.

Level 6: Be Radically Genuine

Act in a manner that communicates respect for the client as a person and an equal, rather than as "client" or "disorder." Play to the person's strengths rather than to fragility, in a manner comparable to how you'd offer help to a treasured colleague or loved one. This is clear-eyed and unflinching—you are what you are and I can handle it and you can handle it. The therapist validates the individual rather than any particular response or behavioral pattern. Kelly Wilson (Wilson & Dufrene, 2009) has talked about this same quality as treating our clients as sunsets, rather than math problems. Rogers and Truax (1967) have described this radically genuine stance:

> He is without front or façade, openly being the feelings and attitudes which at the moment are flowing in him. It involves the element of self-awareness, meaning that the feelings the therapist is experiencing are available to his awareness, and also that he is able to live these feelings, to be them in the relationship, and able to communicate them if appropriate. It means that he comes into a direct personal encounter with his client, meeting him on a person-to-person basis. It means he is being himself, not denying himself. (p. 101)

While empathy and functional validation should remain high throughout therapy, the active verbal validation to provide corrective feedback or to balance pathologizing should be faded from an initially high level early in therapy to normative levels late in therapy. For example, Bettina's parents were highly critical and tended toward the most pathologizing explanation of Bettina's behavior. Early in therapy, the therapist actively offered counterpoints of how Bettina's behavior also was valid. Later in therapy, the therapist expected Bettina to self-validate as well as critique her own behavior in a balanced manner, seeing what is effective and ineffective.

HOW TO USE VALIDATION
TO STRENGTHEN EMOTION REGULATION

Effective emotion regulation requires blending the ability to experience and express emotion (accept emotion) and the ability to actively regulate emotion (change emotion). Les Greenberg writes about this as "emotional wisdom," knowing when to be changed by emotion and when to change emotion (2002, p. xvi).

Prerequisite to either accepting or changing emotion is the ability to identify and label the emotion and make sense of the information the emotion provides. When people have experienced both a lack of validation and pervasive invalidation, they often have significant deficits here (e.g., Ebner-Priemer et al., 2008). Learning to correctly discriminate and label emotions and needs requires caregivers to appropriately attend to those emotions and needs. For example, a 25-year-old client had been raised by a single mother who had been overwhelmed by her own struggles and so self-focused that she never asked questions or noticed much about her daughter (the client). Once the therapist noticed the client's lips looked dry and said, "You look thirsty, would you like some water?" The client had never noticed the sensation of dry lips before nor labeled the internal sensation as "thirsty" (in fact she seldom drank, even with meals).

By using validation strategies, you teach your client to recognize and use his or her experience of emotion (e.g., "Yes, what you are feeling is healthy sadness, it reflects grieving for this important thing you lost" or "Yes, that fear is organizing you to escape this situation that is potentially harmful for you"). This reestablishes the innate, wise-mind, adaptive use of one's own emotional responses to identify what works and is effective. With Mia, for example, validation helps her learn to use anger and its intensity as a signal to identify what need or goal is thwarted and then to choose whether to retaliate (go with the action urge of anger) or to check the facts about the threat and find ways around it to reach her goal or meet her need. Validation strategies can also be used as an informal exposure procedure to strengthen abilities to experience and accept emotion, as well as be used to change emotion by cuing adaptive emotion.

Using Validation as an Informal Exposure Procedure: Accepting Primary Emotions

As discussed in Chapters 1 and 2, the biosocial theory argues that our clients learned that expressing valid needs, emotions, thoughts, or other natural and genuine primary responses brings invalidation. Because these inclinations and responses have been pervasively invalidated, the person learns to avoid his own genuine, primary behavior. In pervasively invalidating environments, fear conditioning takes place so that we not only avoid the feared object (invalidation) but also avoid any experience of the private events (thoughts, sensations, emotions, etc.) which might lead anywhere near invalidation. We become extremely sensitized to all cues that have to do with invalidation *and* we become phobic of our own valid, natural responses. Letting ourselves respond naturally is often as evocative as if you dropped a spider in a spider phobic's lap. Our own primary emotions—those valid first flashes of response—are rapidly followed by escape, that is, a secondary response that ends or modulates the primary response. The avoidance may be subtle. For example, we sense a slight inattention in our therapist as we speak and so we change what we were going to say to a less risky self-disclosure. We feel irritated with our partner without awareness of the more vulnerable first flash of sadness or shame that we rapidly escaped. Escape and avoidance may also be more obvious such as through dissociating in session, or intentional self-injury.

These conditioned emotional reactions and avoidance patterns may come up when you validate or invalidate clients' responses. Consequently, principles of exposure therapy can guide your work. As in more formal use of exposure and response prevention, you identify what specifically cues the difficult emotion(s) and what behaviors function as escape. Then you gradually shape increased emotional experience and expression with cue exposure and response prevention. Over time, with such informal exposures, the client learns to experience and express valid responses with less disruption and less avoidance. It's easiest to see the nuance of this with a clinical example.

One day in session with you, as your client tells you something important about his week, there's an abrupt shift in affect and he looks ashamed. Within a few sentences he is making extreme statements about how he is making no progress, he is a burden to you; he is not using your time well. He looks spacey, and ends with an irritated, "What are we even working on in here?"

The first five times this happened, you went right along with the stated question. Maybe you had an unclear hypothesis about what was going on, a vague sense that he was ashamed. You tried to reduce shame by saying that change is normally often a slow, difficult process. You replied, "Would it be helpful to go back over our goals together and how today's session relates to that?" Now, in this sixth re-run, you realize this scenario plays over and over. Your attempts at reassurance and validation of progress seem to have no effect.

Today, guided by ideas about fear conditioning and exposure therapy, your first move would be to assess what happened that led to the shift, hypothesizing that perhaps a routinized escape pattern has fired. Perhaps shame is a secondary response to a more primary emotion. You ask, "Did something just happen? We were talking about X, then I said Y, and then somewhere you had a big spike in hopeless statements. Can we go back? When I said Y, how did that affect you?" You go microsecond to microsecond to track his experience, using chain analysis to identify the controlling variables of the in-session emotion dysregulation. You learn he began the session glad to see you. The shift was cued when you misunderstood something important he had said.

The first primary flash of emotion was his hurt at being misunderstood. He then instantly judged himself for feeling hurt—he felt ashamed and humiliated to be longing for your understanding. This spiraled into a virulent stream of self-invalidation (the thought "you're an f'ing baby, a bottomless pit") with the theme that he was being immature and over-reactive. Then his anger flared up at the therapist as a primary response to not getting an important need met and at himself as an escape response from these painful, vulnerable emotions. Then he got spacey, irritated that he couldn't focus and irritated with you as nothing therapeutic was happening. You hypothesize that the cue of you misunderstanding him set off a cascade of secondary responses which functioned as escape from the discomfort of *primary emotions* of *longing* (to be understood) and *hurt* (by you misreading him).

It can be hard to sort out what is primary and what is secondary. Greenberg (2002) writes that primary emotions have the quality of shifting in response to the moment's circumstances, feeling fresh or new, feeling whole, deep, and "good" even if not happy. This is in contrast to secondary emotions. When secondary emotions fire, they often obscure or feel diffuse, and the person feels upset, hopeless, confused, or inhibited, and has low energy and is whiney.

With informal exposure then, you would want to re-present the cue. For instance, you might say, "So, when I misunderstood you . . . " When clients are prone to dysregulation, you titrate the presence of the cue to match their tolerance, gradually increasing the intensity of the cue. For example, to gradually intensify the cue for an arachnophobe, starting with pictures of spiders, then moving to having a small spider moving across the room, to eventually handling a tarantula. You are not doing flooding or implosion therapy. To encourage contact and increase tolerance with different private experiences, you provide gentle direction to focus internally—you can instruct the client in the skills of mindfulness of current emotion and of observing and describing emotion. The chain analysis, too, is emotion-focused: you help him put emotions into words, especially encouraging the differentiation and elaboration of primary emotions.

In the above example, the therapist might begin with nearly verbatim paraphrasing of the client and then gently add more intense emotional descriptions of the client's experience as they proceed: "So even though part of you judges your reactions and says it shouldn't bother you, at the same time it *did* bother you. It hurt a little . . . and to me that makes sense, I need and want understanding at moments like that, too" (*Level 5 validation*). A bit further along the therapist validated the emotional need more intensely, still titrating the cue by indirectly validating with a metaphor. "To me emotional needs are like needing water—if I'm crossing the desert and come across a cup of water, it is a big deal. Deprivation naturally makes everything more intense."

The next task in informal exposure is to block avoidance behavior. You help the client experience the primary emotion without escape or other maladaptive coping. The idea is to prevent avoidance responses but to do so in a way that enhances the person's sense of control over the situation and himself. Therefore, before blocking avoidance behaviors, you may explicitly discuss the benefits and drawbacks of avoiding and disrupting primary emotional experience or expression to micro-orient to the rationale to help the client clearly see the benefit of collaborating on the therapy task. As in more formal exposure protocols, you also may ask clients to describe or enact all the ways they avoid (i.e., interrupt or inhibit themselves) when they don't want to feel or express primary emotions or other valid responses. While the ways to avoid emotional experience are myriad, keep your eye out for two common ones that function as escape behaviors. These end contact with emotional experience and thereby disrupt adaptive emotion and other valid behavior: (1) secondary emotions and (2) self-invalidation. Returning to the example above, when you comment that the client felt hurt, you bring him into contact with hurt and disappointment, which gently blocks avoidance. When he then says, "Yeah, but it's silly to feel sad, it was such a small thing" you'd say, "Right, it isn't a huge thing, and yet still it was important to you so you feel a little hurt. I feel hurt, too, when someone misunderstands me on something important." You gently block efforts to escape through habitual self-invalidation, re-present the cue, and validate the primary emotion. Over many such informal exposure interactions, the client increases his tolerance for the painful emotion and engages in less maladaptive avoidance. We can either stay with this until he fully experiences and explores his primary experience of hurt and any action urge that eventually arises from that. Or, if the client has great difficulty experiencing or expressing emotion, even a momentary increase in staying with the experience or expression might best shape approximations toward more regulated emotion.

The final component of informal exposure is to help the client respond differently to primary emotions and other genuine responses. Opposite action is the DBT skill designed to help clients do this. Linehan (1993b) has written about this as literally doing exactly the opposite of the action tendency of the targeted emotion. For example, the action tendency of fear is to freeze or flee. To do the opposite would be to approach. The action urge of shame is to hide and the opposite action would be, for example, to speak openly with upright posture about the "transgression." In the context of using validation as informal exposure, the idea is to stay with, rather than escape, primary emotional experience, and may be even to deliberately lean into the experience instead of pulling away.

However, validation can be incredibly evocative and difficult. Your validating comment about a previously avoided primary emotion or response may increase fear to such an extent that it becomes disruptive and disorganizing. For some clients, validation is actually more difficult to bear than invalidation. Some clients fear that experiencing emotion itself will be traumatic, and they have *in fact experienced* emotions that have overwhelmed them to the point where they have lost control, sometimes in debilitating ways. For example, after a difficult session, a client can't get out of bed for three days. When people have this secondary target of emotion vulnerability, it creates a complex, hard-to-convey blend of shame, despair, desperation, resignation, exhaustion, and an isolating, terrifying certainty that no one can help. For these clients, the trauma associated with emotional experience itself may best be treated by *changing* emotion or skillfully modulating it. Instead of leaning into or deepening emotional experience, the client needs to learn how to move away from emotional experience, but to do so in ways that are not harmful, that accentuate his sense of control, and that diminish the sense of isolation with the experience. One way to help clients develop this ability to change emotion is to use validation to cue adaptive emotion.

Using Validation to Cue Adaptive Emotion: Changing Emotion

Emotions evolved to help us rapidly adapt. Our emotional system constantly registers and rapidly interprets our context, reorganizing and mobilizing us so that our behavior, inclinations, and orientations are constantly shifting to locate and adapt us to our continually changing context. Kelly Wilson's teaching story about the rabbit and the rabbit hole illustrates this process (Wilson & DuFrene, 2008). As a bunny sits on the grassy meadow, he has a full repertoire of behaviors that are possible, some stronger than others. In that sunny, safe context, the bunny eats, looks around, scratches, grooms, lays down. There is a fluid, shifting nature to this responding. But if there is a rustle in the bushes from a predator, those bunnies whose behavioral repertoire narrows to a single response—bolt for the rabbit hole—have considerable survival advantage. In that context, behaviors of stopping for a last scratch or bite to eat become (literally) extinct. Emotionally sensitive bunnies that bolted as soon as they registered the other bunnies' fear also had survival advantage. Emotions work like that according to Greenberg (2002), and emotion theorists like Fridja (1986), Izard (1991); and Tomkins (1963, 1983). We are wired for certain cues to generate complex full-body responses that include rapid assessment of the environment and one's relationship to it, as well as motivation of action and communication to others.

When you validate (or invalidate), you often cue emotion. You can deliberately use this to your client's advantage. When emotion fires it disrupts ongoing activity and organizes the person for the next situation. Using validation to cue adaptive emotion helps activate the entire skillful repertoire associated with the adaptive emotion. In other words, cuing adaptive emotion can rapidly reorganize the client for more adaptive behavior, as shown earlier with Mia. Mia is just like the bunny. She enters the therapy session after the difficult job interview, and she has a whole repertoire of things she can do in session, some more at strength and likely to dominate the moment, others less likely, but all possible and in a meaningful way, *present*, even though not manifest. The therapist's comment to Mia, "That must have been so disappointing!" directs the client's attention and evokes an intensified experience of sadness and disappointment; other disappointing elements of the situation come to mind, followed by tears. When you cue an emotion you cue the *whole* response system that is that emotion. This is as true for adaptive emotions as it is for problematic ones. If you keep this in mind, you can deliberately choose to validate adaptive primary emotions that are present and genuine for the client in a troubling context.

To cue the adaptive emotion, scan for the primary adaptive emotions that are present but in the background of the client's most obvious emotion. This is like being in the forest in a raging windstorm and deliberately listening for the waterfall. Note what the client says yet search for what is also present but less dominant in the person's experience. For example, if someone cuts me off on the freeway, the strongest sensation I feel is anger. But I also feel surprised, disappointed that people drive like that, scared, and humbled as I also at times drive poorly, and so on. If you made a validating comment about any one of these aspects, it would bring me into contact with that part of my experience and likely increase my flexibility: I will not only feel and act angry, but I will also be influenced by whatever else you bring to my attention.

Validating to cue adaptive emotion can't be done as a bait and switch. In other words, if you try to get me off a problematic response by validating something else, it communicates that my primary response is invalid. The trick when scanning for adaptive emotions is to think dialectically, seeing the "truth" in all responses by articulating what is valid about each emotional response. This differentiates the emotions, helping the client have a clearer sense of the action urge and information from his or her emotions. For example, Greenberg (2002) refers to the whining complaint of "why me?" as "the voice of protest" and says this can be thought of as a fused or undifferentiated blend of anger and sadness. Validating to differentiate sadness (e.g., "you are of course terribly disappointed") and irritation (e.g., "what a frustrating situation!") can resolve the experience into a changed emotional and self-organization where the action urge of one emotion becomes more predominant and leads naturally to action.

Cuing adaptive emotion requires the therapist to believe that primary emotion is adaptive and will usefully organize the client. The therapist must resist the temptation to rescue the client from experiencing sadness or despair. Primary emotions are like "a spotlight that turns on to show us what [problem] needs cognition" (Greenberg, 2002). When there is clarity about emotion, its action tendency is naturally harnessed to problem solving.

Emotion "processing" literally takes time. Like potatoes steaming it can't be rushed. But it can be helped. You are looking to strike the right balance between conveying compassion, support, and providing direction. Confirm and focus on what is experienced while offering explicit instructions about how to proceed and new emotional problem-solving strategies. Offer process directions much as you would offer instructions to a new climber on a steep, technically difficult rock face. You can see the next hold, she can't. Tell her where the hold is; instruct her how to shift her weight to her left leg because she's going to have to lunge to reach the hold. You can see the path she needs to take to avoid an impossible reach. There's no use telling her about three holds forward—you provide the instruction as she needs it.

Further, if the climber is panicked, you must somehow reach through the dysregulated state to get her attention. Sometimes the client is so caught in the isolating, dreadful secondary target of emotion vulnerability that he or she fundamentally loses contact with your warmth and support or even at times your presence. Just as the therapist with Mia did in the earlier example, you may need to make certain the client can actually experience your warmth and connection so that you cue enough adaptive emotion to enable collaboration and new learning.

Therefore, when you use validation to cue adaptive emotion, you sometimes travel the high road—strengthening the person's responses in a context where they have been needed but absent, helping to modulate and transform the emotion. When you validate a difficult emotion that's been avoided, it increases contact and acceptance of emotional experience and expression. It may be exactly this shifting from one state to another, bringing disjunctive states together, that is key to transforming maladaptive emotions (Greenberg, 2002). In DBT, you strengthen *both* the ability to effectively change emotion and the ability to accept experience of emotion.

These validation strategies are illustrated in detail in the clinical example that follows. You'll see how the client's attempts to regulate the primary emotion of sadness drives problematic behaviors such as self-invalidation. You'll see different levels of validation, different targets of validation, and the use of validation as informal exposure and a way to cue adaptive emotion.

CASE EXAMPLE: LARA

LARA: I'm hurt and I'm angry and I don't feel like crying about Neal, you know? I'll look like shit, I'll feel worse, you know? So, I don't feel like crying. (*Avoids sadness.*)

THERAPIST: Do you feel worse when you cry? (*Assesses how avoiding sadness may make sense.*)

LARA: No, I just want to be in control, I don't want to be all out of control with everything.

THERAPIST: When you cry, you are out of control? (*Gently challenges the client's perspective that expressing sadness equates to being out of control—the therapist gently invalidates what she views as a maladaptive response.*)

LARA: I'm going to look like shit. I go to work, I look like shit right now. I just want to move on. (*The client responds to the therapist's challenging by intensifying her statement that avoiding expressing sadness is needed.*)

THERAPIST: Do you think you look like shit right now? (*Again challenges the client's view that expressing sadness is problematic and to be avoided.*)

LARA: Yeah, I do. I'm tired, I'm not getting any sleep. It's one o'clock, two o'clock, I have to get up at 7 in the morning. You know? Plus I have to take Neal's stuff back.

THERAPIST: Do you *have* to do that before work? (*Implies this will not be effective for client.*)

LARA: I'm going to do it. (*Voice rises in anger. She feels invalidated—not only that, she was invalidated.*)

THERAPIST: Lara . . . (*Attempts to block escalation by gaining Lara's attention.*)

LARA: I'm going to do it.

THERAPIST: Lara, that's fine if you're going to do it. (*Explicit validation.*) (*Gently.*) I want to help you get through this day. If you want that help, I can give you that help. (*Offers in a tone suggestive of helping the client make genuine choice, not in punitive manner.*) And, what I also want to help you do is not shut off important emotions prematurely because then they keep coming back. (*Orients and cues alternative adaptive emotion of sadness.*)

LARA: (*Cries.*) I've got the wrong makeup on today and it's going to streak all over my face. Why these emotions now, why do I feel like crying? (*Shifts to self-invalidation, a bit of avoidance.*)

THERAPIST: I can think of a lot of reasons you'd feel like crying right now. It seems like a pretty normal response to what's going on, Lara. (*Level 5 validation which sustains contact with cue, sadness, which is usually avoided.*) You've had a lot of sadness and a lot of pain around this, and a lot of hurt. Because you do care about him. (*Again facilitates experience of sadness by validating it.*)

LARA: It's too bad if I care about him. (*Self-invalidation, secondary reaction of anger at self, functions as maladaptive self-regulation of sadness.*)

THERAPIST: OK, hang on. Hang on with me, OK? OK, hang on. (*Blocks escape.*) And what's going on is you're doing it right now—those feelings feel really overwhelming, that sadness, and that feeling of "I don't want to be doing this. I don't want to be out of control." So, your brain flashes to anger. And you feel a little more in control and a little less overwhelmed maybe, with the anger. (*Validates the effectiveness of current thoughts and emotions.*) And so, one way is to try to just stick with the sadness with me for a little while. Then I'll help you put it away in this session and you can go out and do what you need to do, return his stuff, and feel some mastery from doing that. (*Orients.*)

LARA: How can you feel well enough to go to work when you're tired and everything?

THERAPIST: Well you're not going to feel well, but . . .

LARA: I'm going to lose my job. (*For this client, hopelessness is a frequent secondary reaction and functions as avoidance.*)

THERAPIST: That's a hopeless thought, right there. (*Labels to help get distance from the thought and block avoidance.*)

LARA: Well, I will because I am not functioning well. I didn't function Sunday on my job.

THERAPIST: OK, what happened? (*Because the client has had significant problems at work, the therapist has second therapy task here of assessing whether there's a crisis brewing and thus needs to shift the priority of what gets done this session.*)

LARA: I just felt really insecure. I felt hurt, and just like I couldn't get my brain to function or anything.

THERAPIST: OK, now those are three very different things—feeling insecure, not getting your brain to function, and not doing well on the job.

LARA: I didn't feel any sense of self-esteem, the way I used to feel. I don't feel that anymore.

THERAPIST: OK, but do you have any evidence that you didn't actually do well on the job? Or were you just feeling . . .

LARA: The person I worked with was a drag. . . . No, I know my boss loves me, but I can't function!

THERAPIST: OK. (*Decides no crisis is brewing so shifts back to task of experiencing and expressing sadness without attendant avoidance.*) That's what I want to help you with because I think if you spend a little bit of time with the sadness, that would help you regulate it so you are not overwhelmed. (*Reorients to the task of informal exposure to facilitate emotion regulation.*) See what happens is, you get close to it and then you run away from it—you never have a chance to get past it.

LARA: I'm crying now, aren't I?

THERAPIST: You are crying now. (*Gently.*) So you're feeling a lot of hurt.

LARA: Yeah.

THERAPIST: Yeah. Tell me about that. (*Level 1 validation functions to re-present the cue to extend informal exposure.*)

LARA: Well, the hurt is a realization that the man is really sick and I cannot be with him. I will not be with him.

THERAPIST: And how do you feel when you think about not being with him? (*Gentle pressure to keep focusing on sadness.*)

LARA: I feel sad, but at the same time I feel a sense of relief, too.

THERAPIST: Do you? You feel both?

LARA: Yes.

THERAPIST: And what else comes up when you think about not being with him? (*Continues gentle pressure to keep focusing on sadness.*)

LARA: Loneliness.

THERAPIST: Yeah.

LARA: I'm not worth anything as a woman.

THERAPIST: Yeah.

LARA: You know?

THERAPIST: Yeah, let's stick with that a moment. (*Senses that loneliness is important primary emotion, likely adaptive, and directs attention to this.*)

LARA: Which is not true. I know, I know I can get better than him.

THERAPIST: um hmm. So, this is the sort of thing that you do to try to keep those feelings under control . . . to tell yourself you know it'll get better. (*Highlights secondary response of cognitive counterevidence.*) And you know what you're saying is not true, so OK.

LARA: I'm being real careful not to turn the anger on myself, which is part of what happens with women who stay with men who are bad for them.

THERAPIST: So let's stick with the loneliness, OK—not with the other, there's no one really. (*Again re-presents cue for loneliness.*)

LARA: I've got friends. (*Avoids.*)

THERAPIST: OK, so we're talking about men. (*Again re-presents cue for loneliness.*)

LARA: I've been asked out on dates. I was asked out the next night. (*Avoids.*)

THERAPIST: OK now.

LARA: That's not a problem, but I don't want to date anybody right now.

THERAPIST: OK, what I'm doing is trying to . . . (*Blocks avoidance and now orients to increase Lara's collaboration and insight into the pattern.*)

LARA: But you're going to look at it differently.

THERAPIST: Yeah, it seems like the thought of loneliness is so scary that you've got to say "but I've got dates. . . . " It's difficult to just stick to the fact that maybe you'll be alone. Maybe you'll feel lonely.

LARA: Yeah, but I won't forever.

THERAPIST: You may not. But do you follow what I'm saying? I'm trying to . . .

LARA: . . . get me to accept the fact that I feel lonely.

THERAPIST: And the reason for that is . . . I think that's a very scary thing for you.

LARA: Yeah.

THERAPIST: And it starts triggering all these thoughts and all these behaviors, like calling Neal. The whole thing with fear is we need to confront what we're afraid of to get over that fear. So, sometimes it is real good to tell yourself it's not going to last, it's going to change. But right now I want you not to do that. I want you to just experience being alone and being lonely and whatever comes up with that. To know that you can experience that and move on without having to run from it.

LARA: OK.

THERAPIST: OK, so right now Neal is out of your life. (*Resumes presenting cue of loneliness and encouraging experience.*)

LARA: Yes.

THERAPIST: There's not anyone else. Even if you've got people calling you, there's not anyone that really knows you, really cares about you yet, and there may not be . . .

LARA: Well, there's Mario.

THERAPIST: Yeah, he's married.

LARA: Yeah, he's only a friend.

THERAPIST: Yeah, only a friend—so that's different. (*Again the therapist views loneliness as a key emotion, so, she re-presents the cues associated with loneliness to help better differentiate the emotions.*)

LARA: Even though I feel like that, it's not really . . .

THERAPIST: So, what's coming up when you think about lonely is a lot of statements about . . .

LARA: My worth.

THERAPIST: So, what's the feeling associated with that?

LARA: Another failed relationship.

THERAPIST: "Another failed relationship," "I can't . . . " what? (*Attempts to further assess what's most painful and avoided.*)

LARA: Well, I shouldn't think those thoughts. (*Self-invalidates.*)

THERAPIST: But, wait a minute. You *should* think those thoughts right now, OK, because those are the thoughts that come into your head (*Level 5 validation.*) So, you keep trying to . . . is this what you normally do? You say, "I shouldn't think those thoughts, and . . . (*Begins to highlight the way these secondary reactions function as avoidance.*)

LARA: Well, if I think despairing thoughts, I'm going to feel despairing . . .

THERAPIST: Right.

LARA: I don't want to think that. It'll pull me down. (*Wants to avoid despair, a primary maladaptive emotion for her that is extremely difficult and a link to intentional self-injury and suicidal behavior. In other words, "know thy client."*)

THERAPIST: Right, I think what we're doing is going to help that.

LARA: Why?

THERAPIST: Because we're exposing you to the feelings that come up with these thoughts. The feelings keep coming back, because you say things like "I shouldn't think that way," but the problem is you *are* thinking that way. So the solution is not to say "I shouldn't think that way." I mean, you don't want to think hopeless thoughts and dwell and dwell. But you get these emotions that come up as a result of loss, not just from the thoughts, and then you think thoughts to cope with that. (*Level 5 validation orients.*)

LARA: Like "I shouldn't feel this way."

THERAPIST: Right.

LARA: I shouldn't feel a sense of loss.

THERAPIST: Right. So, I want to stay with one thought that's really big for you, which is "I'm not worth anything." What's the feeling that comes up with that thought? (*Again returns to gentle focus on emotional experience.*)

LARA: Shame.

THERAPIST: Shame. Can you feel that now, while we're talking?

LARA: Yeah, shameful and guilty.

THERAPIST: OK, let's stay focused on your feelings. We know he triggers a lot of those feelings. We know it's a given.

LARA: I'm just so used to feeling ashamed and I berate myself, judge myself. Like I called him the other day, and then I think, that totally undermines my credibility. If it's as bad as I say it is why am I calling him. That's crazy. I'm exaggerating the whole thing.

THERAPIST: OK, so wait, that's what happens right? It's happening right now. You felt lonely and called him, then you judge yourself. How could you do something different right there? Let's just take that: you shouldn't have called Neal.

LARA: I could say, "So I called Neal. It's not the end of the world. I made a mistake." I've read that rational-emotive therapy.

THERAPIST: And it seems like you have been practicing that some. When I was trying to get you to stay with an emotion you were coming back with thoughts to kind of change that emotion. So it seems like that's a skill you have. What you want to be careful with, though, is to use it wisely. Don't try to cut off your emotion really quickly all the time. Unless you need to cut it off right away—like you need to go to work, for example. Is there a way that you don't have to invalidate it? Like what you said right there: "OK, I called him. I made a mistake." I might not say . . .

LARA: You don't have to be upset about it (*self-invalidation*).

THERAPIST: But you *do* feel upset. See, that's what you have to be really careful about with changing your thoughts. You don't want to invalidate your feelings in the process. So, maybe instead, could we try this— (*Notes time left in session, knows the client's experiencing and expression in this session were very high for her and now wants to help the client more actively regulate in preparation for winding down the session.*) Could it be that you feel the upset, the guilt? Yes? You don't want to invalidate a single one. You may soothe yourself a little bit by saying, "OK, I feel guilty about this, I feel a lot of emotions, that's OK, that is totally normal, hard but normal. I can move through this, feel what I feel, and take good care of myself." Let's start to look at how you can observe and describe emotions today, OK, and then do self-soothing and self-validation. Let's get a plan of how to get through today without having to push away and escape the emotion, OK? (*Offers skills that will replace self-invalidation and foster emotional experience while moderating intensity of emotion.*)

In this example, the therapist uses validation strategies to strengthen the client's ability to regulate emotion. The dialogue begins with the client hurt and angry. Using validation as informal exposure, the therapist helps the client to experience and express the primary emotion of first sadness and then loneliness and blocks the client's habitual use of self-invalidation to manage overwhelming emotion. There are also change strategies (as described in Chapter 3) woven throughout this dialogue such as micro-orienting. The therapist also shifts gears briefly to assess whether a higher-priority target (job difficulties) might need to be addressed but decides that treating this link of accepting difficult emotions and helping the client practice this in session will best ward off crises that come from the client's more habitual ways of escaping painful emotions.

In general, when a client is dysregulated, I validate problem importance, task difficulty, emotional pain, the sense of being out of control, the wisdom in the client's ultimate goals, and in particular the client's location perspective. Remember to search for the valid; "know thy client"; validate the valid, and invalidate the invalid; and validate at the highest possible level, based on Linehan's levels of validation.

Precise validation with people who are exquisitely sensitive to invalidation can be difficult, and therefore is among the most essential abilities to cultivate as a DBT therapist. In DBT, you balance acceptance-oriented validation strategies and change oriented strategies to match the client's actual vulnerabilities as you benevolently demand needed change. Developing a stance of holding seemingly contradictory elements in mind at the same time is the focus of the next chapter on Dialectics. Dialectics helps the therapist cultivate the capacity of unwavering centeredness needed to bear the intense pain our clients experience and to bear, too, the knowledge that we sometimes inadvertently or unavoidably add to the pain, even as we help the client change to alleviate suffering.

FIVE

Dialectical Stance and Strategies

Balancing Acceptance and Change

The test of a first-rate intelligence is the ability to hold two opposed ideas in the mind at the same time and still retain the ability to function. One should, for example, be able to see that things are hopeless and yet be determined to make them otherwise.
—F. SCOTT FITZGERALD, *The Crack-Up* (1936)

When clients have complex, life-threatening problems that evoke high emotion, our work requires us to think clearly in extreme circumstances. Yet in the face of complexity or ambiguity, when the stakes are high, we grab for the certainty of old patterns and become less psychologically flexible. Clients and therapists become polarized and get into power struggles.

The dialectical stance and strategies in DBT provide a practical means to regain and retain psychological flexibility and balance so that therapeutic movement is possible. DBT's emphasis on freedom, balance, and skillful means comes from Linehan's study of Zen; in fact, dialectical behavior therapy was almost called Zen behavior therapy (Linehan, personal communication, 1990). This third and final set of DBT's core strategies involves the ability to resist oversimplification and move beyond feeble or precarious compromises to find genuinely workable combinations of problem-solving and validation, reason and emotion, acceptance and change.

The therapist "is dialectical" or "acts dialectically" in two ways. First, he or she takes a dialectical stance, embraces a worldview in which he or she can simultaneously hold the positions of accepting the client and the moment completely as they are and moving urgently toward change. He or she views polarization as natural, knowing that a workable truth evolves from looking for validity in each element and for the whole that encompasses them. The therapist moves to and from this dialectical stance whenever therapy comes to an impasse in order to make sense of and respond to ambiguity and conflict. Second, he or she uses particular strategies dialectically. These include the change and validation strategies covered in Chapters 3 and 4, as well as stylistic case management, and specific dialectical strategies described later in this chapter. Returning to dialectics, both stance and strategies, again and again, can keep your mind agile and flexible.

DIALECTICAL STANCE

Taking a dialectical stance is the psychological equivalent of taking a physically centered stance. Your stance determines what moves are possible. If you hunker down, wide-legged, and rooted, it is hard to pirouette. If you shift all of your weight onto the ball of one foot, it is hard to push with any power, but it might be the only way to reach an outstretched hand. Taking a centered stance, however, makes it possible to move flexibly, to reach, push, or pirouette. To counter the way our minds typically become rigid or tiptoe around in conflict, a dialectical stance means adopting a set of assumptions that create a center of psychological flexibility. They let you move freely to match the moment.

Three assumptions define DBT's dialectical stance: (1) reality is whole and interrelated; (2) reality is complex and in polarity; and (3) change is continual and transactional. Taken together they allow you to move flexibly when faced with ambiguity, contradiction, or conflict.

Reality Is Whole and Interrelated

First, a dialectical perspective holds that the nature of reality is holistic, connected, and in relationship. We talk *as if* parts are somehow separate and independent of the whole, yet we simultaneously recognize this is only a manner of speaking. We can only tell something is an element or part because of its connected relationship to the whole. Consider a simple example like a basketball game. We might talk as if the behavior of a given individual player is independent, yet the individual's behavior is determined by the whole. When the teams play a man-to-man defense, the defender tracks the opponent closely to guard against a shot. The connections are obvious; a change in player *A* leads to a change in player *B*. As the ball moves, so do the players. Each player's move connects directly to an opponent's. Sometimes the connection of a part to the whole is less obvious, more like a zone defense, where one player's shifting position leads to some change but not as much as in a man-to-man matchup.

Similarly, when we make this assumption of holistic interdependence in therapy, we may still talk *as if* therapist and client are separate and independent yet when we look deeply we see they are connected and are part of a larger whole. From this view, separateness and simplistic linear causality are less dominant, even considered misperception. A Zen teaching example illustrates this well. A Zen master might hold a sheet of ordinary paper and ask, "What is this?" "Paper," we'd say. Wood pulp and the chemicals used to make pulp. Years of sunshine and rain that fed the trees that make the pulp. Light particles that came from distant stars; water molecules that came from distant seas. The workers, who harvested the trees, pulped and made the paper, packaged and brought it to the store. All the connections that led to the workers being able to do those tasks: others who grew and prepared their food; others who designed and created each machine used. We see that the piece of paper contains the entire universe in a quite literal way. The sheet of paper can be said to be entirely "nonpaper elements," an instant of many causal processes coming together in a particular space and time that is labeled at that instant "paper." The same might be said of the discrete space and time we call "therapist" or "client."

We see this but lose our understanding of interdependence when faced with ambiguity and conflict. When a client does something we dislike (e.g., leaves an attacking phone message, demands help we cannot give), our conditioned first response is for our attention to narrow into a static sense of The Other doing something to Me that must be fixed or avoided. We lose track of the fact that the client's behavior is as much the coming together of many causal strands as is the piece of paper. All the circumstances required to cause this moment to arise have in fact occurred. Our own response of irritation, our evaluative labels of "problematic" or "inappropriate" are also the result of many conditions coming together. For example, given different professional training, we might be delighted (rather than irritated) when clients do with us what happens elsewhere in life—we get to work directly on it.

This assumption that reality is whole, related, and in connection, leads to seeing that everything is caused, and therefore in a profound sense could not be otherwise. Both client and therapist responses are equally caused, even when we can't see the causal web. This means that from a dialectical perspective, assessment and intervention take into account not only the client but also the relationships among the client, the client's community, the therapist, and the therapist's community. For example, in the West we tend to locate pathology in the patient. With dialectical views, assessment is instead directed to the whole system. For example, one client's extreme sensitivity was at least in part due to the extreme invalidation of racism he experienced. His very dark skin and large size made everyday tasks like standing in a grocery checkout a gauntlet of invalidation as people unconsciously moved to stand further from him or the clerk involuntarily startled and recoiled with her first glance. Informed by dialectical philosophy, the therapist and treatment team strive to view the person in context, particularly turning to search the greater causal web to see what is left out of the case formulation when there is an impasse (dialectical assessment).

Reality Is Complex and in Polarity

Second, a dialectical perspective holds that reality is complex, oppositional, and in polarity. Again, we intuitively recognize this from our lives and clinical work. Say a 12-year-old runaway (built like a 15-year-old) is admitted to a psychiatric unit by police. The file shows he's had horrible physical abuse as a child and mild developmental disability. As you interview him he appears to have manic symptoms with extreme irritability. Multiple drugs show in the tox screen. He's admitted for observation. At this point you think, "Huh, there is this and there is that, and then there is this other piece, wow, this is complicated." But then he physically threatens the petite, beloved social worker in a sexually graphic way; now there is high emotion among the staff. As soon as someone on the inpatient unit takes the position of being flexible on program rules, it elicits someone else's description of why in this case no exceptions to the rule should be made. One person thinks the client can be reasonably discharged, which prompts someone else on the team to give reasons why that is not a good idea. We often respond to complexity in oppositional or polarized ways. The existence of "yes" gives rise to "no"; "all" to "nothing." Maybe it is the nature of reality or maybe simply the nature of human perception or language. Whatever the reason, we often fall into processes in which oppositional elements are in tension with each other. When applied to human conflict, often both opposing positions may be true or contain elements of the truth (e.g., there are valid reasons to discharge *and* to delay discharge). Taken together, these first two dialectical assumptions mean no one ever has a "whole" perspective on a client. Therapists are like the blind men each touching a part of an elephant and each being certain that the whole is exactly as the part they are touching. "An elephant is big and floppy," "no, no, long and round and thin," "no, no, no, solid like a wall." Each has an alternative perspective. Each is true and each is partial.

From this view, then, smart, reasonable people will disagree. Polarized divergent opinions are seen as inevitable when problems are complex. Nothing is wrong: the client isn't pathologically splitting the team; the therapist isn't (necessarily) naïve or narcissistic. It is simply the nature of the phenomenon. No one person on a treatment team has a lock on the truth. Any understanding is likely partial and missing something important. Therefore, DBT puts a large emphasis on dialogues that lead to synthesis. How does the piece I hold fit with yours to make a more complete, coherent, or workable whole? Together we search for what is valid in polarized or divergent positions rather than striving for a unified front. Rather than artificially resolve a conflict by dropping one end of the dialectic or fighting only for one (my!) position, effort is made to stay engaged without appeasing, capitulating, dominating, or accepting the invalid.

Change Is Continual and Transactional

Third, a dialectical perspective holds that, if you look deeply, change is continual even though it may be so incremental it is hard to notice. A seed placed in the ground is in constant change—swelling, germinating, growing into a flower and decaying to become the nutrients that nourish the next seed. Despite this continual change, our predominant experience is of continuity. We experience the continuity of our physical bodies, when in fact all the molecules in our bodies have changed. These incremental changes at times coalesce in sudden change. A concrete overpass freezes and thaws, infinitesimally changing with each truck and car until suddenly it fails and collapses. The assumption here is that the whole of nature is in motion: you can never step in the same river twice (Heraclitus). Our minds see mostly unchanging continuity, but from a dialectical perspective, continual change is more primary. The impression of static continuity is an artifact or misperception.

Identity, too, is seen as relational and in continuous change. The only reason he looks old is because she looks younger; the only reason I look rigid is because you are flexible. If a new, more rigid person joins our team then, suddenly, I look quite flexible by comparison. Taking a dialectical perspective means that words like "good" or "bad" or "dysfunctional" are snapshots of the person in context, not qualities inherent in the person. My favorite examples come from watching consultation teams or skills training groups over time. Someone is always "a problem." Whoever happens to be the most (pick your adjective: negative/positive, task-focused/process-focused) drives the rest of us crazy. Yet, if people are forced to stay in the situation, something always happens and they change, sometimes radically. Once in a skills training group a client was "a problem," offering constant negative comments and harsh but whip-smart criticism. By contrast, the lead skills trainer looked like a defensive Pollyanna. When a new co-trainer rotated into the skills group, he shared the same style of sarcastic humor as "the problem client," but instead of being harsh, he had a delightful, wry smile. He admired and was fond of the lead skills trainer. The group chemistry turned criticism into banter and created a lighter but still pointed feedback loop. Released from the siege mentality and genuinely seeing the humor in it all now, the group leader became more creative and likable herself. The "problem client" had less to criticize and could learn more easily. Things settled down (until the next "problem" person arose!).

Dialectics in Balancing Goals

Maintaining a dialectical stance can be hard for therapists because the pull is to become locked into a concept at either end of the pole rather than directly experience how two truths stand side by side as part of a larger synthesis. This can be particularly difficult for two of DBT's main goals— enhancing client emotion regulation and decreasing priority targets such as self-injury. For this reason, DBT therapists view both these goals in dialectical terms.

Dialectics of Emotion Regulation

DBT proposes a dialectical goal regarding emotion regulation. Clients learn skills to change emotion and to accept emotion as it is. In the abstract, these positions seem contradictory, a mixed message about how to respond to private experience. Yet if we examine our actual experience, the paradox resolves. The most difficult moments of our lives often require both downregulating (changing) and mindfully experiencing (accepting) our emotional responses.

Consider a clinical example. A client, in bitter divorce proceedings, lost primary custody of her 2-year-old daughter. The husband's lawyer built a humiliating account of her repeated psychiatric hospitalizations and suicide attempts, successfully negating her more recent treatment progress. Anyone would feel anguished at losing custody, especially when one's own transgressions contributed to the decision. However, for this client, her emotions were at an unrelenting, all-consuming intensity. She was crazed with pain. Contact with her ex-husband, both in real life and in imagination, was like a match to gasoline. Her pain would ignite into rage and revenge fantasies. She loathed herself, certain that his claim she was a terrible mother was true and her daughter would be better off without her. She sobbed, grief-stricken each time she imagined a future without living day to day with her daughter. She had urges to capitulate and give up visitation rather than endure the pain. She sat in shock, detached and numb for hours.

She had little time, however, to sort out these feelings to inform her next set of actions because the court required that she begin mediation to determine visitation privileges. To establish credibility and best negotiate terms for visitation the client needed to demonstrate her competence. In these emotionally challenging interactions with the court or her ex-husband, her mind was in an uproar. Yet if she displayed even a whiff of emotion dysregulation, her husband would use it against her. Her goals in the situation demanded exquisite emotion regulation.

Based on the chain analysis, the therapist and client identified shame as the primary emotion that led to the most escaping into problematic responding. This was especially the case when the client heard or thought she was "a bad mother." In one extended session, the client and therapist looked in an unflinching way at how this criticism was true: that is, the client listed all the ways she had failed her daughter and failed to meet her own standards. The therapist, as described in the last chapter, used validation to hold the client in informal exposure episodes so that she could experience shame without escaping into problematic secondary responses. Validation also cued adaptive emotion: the reason for her hurt and shame was how desperately she loved and wanted the best for her daughter, how terribly she longed to be a good mother. The client and therapist practiced the DBT skill of radical acceptance, looking at the causal web that created all the conditions that led to the failings as a mother, without sugarcoating the harm the client had done. Both spontaneously and with the therapist's help, the client experienced how shame transformed into deep regret and the healthy action urge to make amends and repair the damage. She found a kernel of pride at how fiercely she was using this therapy to change to do better by her daughter.

The client also struggled with rage at her husband. Here the therapist helped the client actively downregulate anger and avoid anger cues in order to avoid physically or verbally attacking her husband or his property (which she had done many times in the past). For example, the client's friends loyally sided with her, and fueled her anger by doing things like using the husband's picture as a dartboard, plotting to ruin his reputation at work, and talking endlessly about how unfair he had been. In the lead up to the mediation meeting, the client recruited her friends to change tactics with her: they either talked about the circumstances in a completely low-key nonjudgmental manner (e.g., "divorces are really hard," "there are things about this situation I don't like") or they avoided the topic and focused on areas where the client was building a new life.

Further, the client and therapist identified the two most anger-provoking things the husband did and practiced drills where the therapist presented the cues and the client deliberately altered her breathing to calm herself. She inhaled for a count of 3, held her breath for a count of 2, then exhaled for 5, slowly and fully, pausing for 2 counts at the end of the exhalation. In this practice, she actively imagined picking up each thought or emotion about her situation and putting it in a box, gently saying "later." She practiced this exercise and radical acceptance of shame on her own while gazing at a picture of her husband holding their daughter. She repeatedly put the picture into an envelope and then brought it out again to gaze at the picture and practice. The client learned how to control her attention in order to make fuller contact with emotion cues. She also learned to distract from emotion cues in order to down-regulate emotion. From a dialectical perspective, both approaches are valid and the focus was to help the client discriminate when either strategy did or did not fit her goals in the moment.

Dialectical Abstinence

Dialectical abstinence is another typical DBT goal that holds two seemingly contradictory elements in one view. The therapist asks the client to commit to stop the problem behavior (e.g., using drugs or intentional self-injury) immediately and permanently, without exception. The therapist adopts an unrelenting insistence on total abstinence, one moment at a time. The message conveyed is that engaging in the problem behavior again would be disastrous. Simultaneously, if a lapse occurs, the therapist takes a nonjudgmental, problem-solving approach to relapse prevention. Like Marlatt's (Marlatt and Donovan, 2005) prolapse strategy, the intention is to minimize "the abstinence violation effect." After a lapse, we often feel intense negative emotions and thoughts (e.g., "What's the point? I've already blown it. I might as well really go for it.") that can interfere with reestablishing abstinence. When there is a lapse, the therapist who is using a dialectical approach helps the client identify factors that led to the lapse in order to devise a plan to prevent such lapses in the future. Then the therapist asks for a recommitment to total abstinence.

By analogy, dialectical abstinence is like climbing an icy trail to safety when lost in a snowstorm. You may die if you don't keep climbing. Any slip can be life threatening. Therefore 100% of your energy is put into staying on your feet and moving. Yet if you fall, you get up. You get directly back to putting 100% of your energy toward moving forward and not falling. If you are a surgeon, the same is true with nicking arteries. You put 100% attention to flawless technique; and if you make a mistake, you repair it quickly. Then 100% of attention is back to the task.

DIALECTICALLY BALANCING STRATEGIES

Using strategies dialectically keeps the therapy moving through impasse. I've already discussed how validation strategies are dialectically balanced with behavioral strategies such as orienting, commitment, chain analysis, and problem solving. Three other important strategy sets are used dialectically to prevent rigid polarization: stylistic strategies, case management strategies, and specific dialectical strategies. Stylistic strategies offer a practical dialectic in how the therapist communicates, balancing being warmly reciprocal and irreverently confrontive. Case management strategies concern how the therapist helps the client to navigate his or her social environment, balancing consulting to the client with direct intervention on the client's behalf in some limited cases. Specifically, dialectical strategies directly target polarization. In each case, the aim is to create the appropriate mix of acceptance of the client's vulnerability and change that recognizes the client's strengths.

Stylistic Strategies: Reciprocal and Irreverent

In DBT, the therapist balances two communication styles: reciprocal and irreverent. A reciprocal communication style emphasizes acceptance. The therapist is sensitive to the nuance in the client's behavior, takes the client's agenda seriously and directly responds to it rather than interpreting any latent meaning. If a client asks something personal about the therapist, the therapist, responding in a reciprocal style, is likely to use self-disclosure, warm engagement, and genuineness to answer the question. A reciprocal style can also be used to matter-of-factly decline to answer based on the therapist's professional or personal limits. From this style, the therapist may use self-disclosure to help the client understand how the client's behavior affects the therapist, to model, or to validate. Such strategic disclosures can enhance the therapeutic relationship, normalize clients' experiences, model adaptive and intimacy building behavior (Goldfried, Burckell, & Eubanks-Carter, 2003), demonstrate genuineness (Robitschek & McCarthy, 1991), equalize power in the therapeutic relationship (Mahalik, Van Ormer, & Simi, 2000), enhance the therapeutic relationship, and establish it as more similar to outside relationships, thus facilitating generalization (Tsai et al., 2008).

However, a reciprocal communication style alone or an imbalance toward this style can lead to impasse. When the glum client who has told the same story of grievance many times has a therapist who simply paraphrases in the same monotone as the client, the probability is that the client's mood will stay the same or worsen. Emotionally intense clients have often had others tiptoe around them as a way to prevent or dampen their emotionality. Consequently, the person never gets needed feedback about problems. For these reasons, reciprocal communication is balanced with an irreverent style that emphasizes change.

Irreverent communication includes using humor or reframing a client's communication in an unorthodox or offbeat manner. Irreverent communication also includes: plunging in where angels fear to tread, oscillating the intensity of emotional tone or language, expressing impotence or omnipotence, using a confrontational tone, and calling the client's bluff. To *plunge in where angels fear to tread* means the therapist says, with a plain-spoken, matter-of-fact manner, what others avoid saying. For example, to the woman who cuts herself when her husband threatens to leave her, "look, cutting yourself and leaving blood all over the bathroom is destroying any hope of having a real relationship with your husband." Or to a new client, "Given that you've assaulted two of your three last therapists, let's start off with what led up to that and how it's not going to happen with me. I'm going to be of no use to you if I'm afraid of you."

A therapist may *oscillate intensity*. The therapist, who has been just as engaged as the client in a power struggle, suddenly shifts tone and laughs, "You know, this moment is just not as black-and-white as I had hoped." A highly suicidal client knows he needs to stay active on weekends to avoid long stretches of unstructured time. He and the therapist begin to brainstorm. As the therapist becomes increasingly active, the client becomes increasingly passive. With remarkable aim, the client shoots down each idea as unfeasible or too inconvenient. At a moment of impasse, the therapist might oscillate intensity by shifting forward in his chair, and with an urgent, intense quiet voice says, "This is life-and-death. Your life is falling apart. If we can't find a way for me to win this power struggle to get you more active, you may die." Or instead at that same impasse the therapist might *express impotence*:

THERAPIST: Well, bummer. That was my last idea. (*Long pause.*) My mind's blank. (*Sits silently for a full minute following his breath.*)

CLIENT: Don't give up, I need help.

THERAPIST: (*Sighs.*) I know, those were my best ideas. I don't have any more.

The client then had room to suggest ideas. On the flip side, the therapist may *express omnipotence*. For example, to a client who is arguing she's too defective and has no "wise mind," the therapist might say, "No, I know these things—you have a wise mind."

Using an irreverent style of communication can include *using a confrontational tone*. A client had a history of many interpersonal problems due to poorly regulated anger. She came to session angry with her therapist for failing to return a phone call promptly. As she entered the therapy office, she launched into her complaint, rapidly raising her voice loud enough to disturb the people in the next office. The therapist used a confrontational tone, saying firmly and loudly, "Stop talking." The client, startled, did stop. The therapist continued, "You are starting to yell and this is too important." The client began to speak, and the therapist interrupted, "No. Listen to me (and then he dropped into a quietly urgent voice, barely above a whisper) this is too important. I *want* to hear what has upset you. When you yell, I can't hear you. I want to hear you. Sit down, tell me about the problem, but don't yell. OK?" The therapist used a confrontational tone as well as off-the-wall reframing when her client, a phlebotomist, threatened to leave a vial of her blood in an ex-lover's inbox at work: "That's old mental patient behavior. I thought we were past that." The client, stung, paused. The therapist continued, changing to a reciprocal tone, "When are you going to take yourself seriously? You loved him so much and you are hurting, that is legitimate. You need comforting, not all this dramatic distraction. I know you are so hurt."

Clients also use irreverent communication when at an impasse. A client felt her therapist was pulling her to change and she was resisting because he kept oversimplifying the problem. It felt like a tug-of-war, each pulling with all their might. Suddenly she dropped her side of the argument, much as you might drop your end of the rope in tug-of-war. She suddenly shifted back in her chair and said with her best smart-ass smile, "Isn't there some kind of an acronym you should be using here?" It so caught the therapist off guard that he laughed. He shifted to her bantering tone.

THERAPIST: Yes. IMHO. "In My Humble Opinion."

CLIENT: I haven't learned that one yet, do they teach that in skills group?

THERAPIST: No. It's a skill some clients teach to their therapists when there is not a two-by-four handy.

Both therapist and client laughed.

Calling the patient's bluff is the most difficult irreverent strategy to describe because the therapist must be exquisitely sensitive to the client's capabilities and context so as not to push her into further extreme statements and instead create a way for her to retract an extreme statement without feeling humiliated. For example, a client from a well-to-do family had learned to respond to unwelcome limits imposed in past therapies with belligerent threats to fire the therapist or report the therapist to his supervisor. Over the course of her second session of individual therapy in her new DBT program, she told her therapist she would need to bring her therapy dog to skills group, the therapist must agree that he would not seek information from her prior therapists, and that she needed him to immediately put a planned admission agreement into place with a specific hospital. The therapist assumed that these requests had some validity and began gently questioning the client so he could understand what was important to her. She rapidly escalated in defensiveness and threats, and within moments had stormed out of the room saying she was going to quit the program. The client then left the therapist 20 increasingly desperate and demanding messages over the course of the afternoon. The therapist called the client back to kindly and respectfully explain that he would appreciate meeting at her earliest convenience, that he never tackled such important questions over the phone. She agreed. When they met the next day, in a completely unflappable deadpan manner, he said he genuinely thought he could be of help, he had no doubt her needs were valid, and that he would be happy to creatively problem solve within his personal and professional limits if she would like. He acknowledged her perfect right to make whatever decisions she saw fit, including firing him or complaining about him. Without fanfare he set a list of his supervisors' names and phone numbers all the way up to the center's CEO near her elbow on the table as he began accurately paraphrasing each of her valid concerns he'd noted in the prior meeting. His unwaveringly centered manner created a pathway for her to engage without further extreme behavior.

You shift your weight from reciprocal to irreverent styles and back in order to keep forward momentum on therapy tasks. For example, a client, prone to anxious rumination, began to describe how disturbed he was by a comment he had learned that his supervisor had made about him. In a meeting with all the county administrators, the client's supervisor had said that he (the client) "smelled bad." The therapist gave a genuine sound of shared pain (reciprocal style), and then reframed in an unorthodox off-beat manner, "Oh, ouch! Yuck!" Then with a little twinkle in her eye, said, "But I gotta say, that's not half as bad as the things you've said about her to some of those same people." The client guffawed in acknowledgment. Irreverence shifted him completely away from his typical downward spiral into anxious rumination. With a sense of humor, he then recalled and exaggerated some of the criticisms he'd made publicly about his supervisor, and then shifted into a more proactive stance. He and the therapist began to problem solve what, if any, action made sense in the circumstance. The therapist shifted back into a warm, engaged, and responsive style, actively validating the client's emotional responses as the client discussed the pros and cons of letting the comment go versus taking some action. (This supervisor had made many inappropriate comments about her supervisees in that meeting, including a racial slur.) The client settled on an email documenting his concerns. The therapist helped by jotting down notes to help the client remember his key points, and then, writing with large loopy handwriting, said, "Yes, and then let's sign it, 'Love, Stinky.'" Both client and therapist laughed until they cried. Reciprocal communication is balanced by irreverence that jolts the person off track to enable the client to resume the therapeutic task.

Case Management Strategies

People in the client's social and professional network often don't know what the client can and cannot do without help. They treat the client as fragile and step in to control when in fact the client is capable, or they expect performance beyond the client's true capability and fail to offer needed help. When multiple treatment providers as well as family or friends are actively involved in clients' lives and treatment, conflict becomes more likely. Often these important others have strong opinions about what should and should not be done in therapy and want to discuss with the therapist what can be done about the identified patient. In DBT these common problems are addressed by balancing the change-oriented intervention of "consultation to the client" with acceptance-oriented environmental intervention. Consultation to the client helps the client become more skillful in personal and professional relationships. In environmental intervention, the therapist accepts the client's true vulnerability and so directly and actively intervenes on the client's behalf.

Consultation to the Client

The spirit of DBT is to address the client's vulnerability by actively helping to remedy skills deficits. Therefore, the DBT therapist's default position is to consult to the client on how to be skillful with others, rather than to intervene with other treatment providers and loved ones about how to deal with the client. You teach the client to skillfully speak for him- or herself across these relationships. While using consultation-to-the-client strategies, the DBT therapist may give other professionals general information about the patient's care; however, details are not discussed without the patient present, preferably with the client himself leading the conversation. In the consulting role the therapist does not tell others how to treat the client, does not intervene or solve problems for the client with other professionals, and does not defend other professionals. Instead, the therapist teaches the client to act as his or her own agent in obtaining appropriate care and maintaining good relationships with realistic expectations.

For example, when a client complained that a skills group leader was covering the material too quickly and treating her (the client) as an irritatingly slow learner, the therapist consulted to the client about what she wanted to do. Would the client rather work on changing the skills trainer or work on her ability to tolerate someone being impatient with her, or both? The individual therapist keeps this spirit of consultation to the client even within the DBT team. Continuing the example above, the individual therapist did not ask the skills trainer to better pace the teaching for her client or express less irritation toward her client. Instead, after consulting to her client, the individual therapist said that her client was having some difficulty in group and that she was coaching the client on how to use both interpersonal skills and distress tolerance. The skills group leaders might expect a call from the client to request a meeting because the client wanted to discuss how she could get more from the group.

Even in a crisis, the spirit of consulting to the client is maintained whenever possible. If a client goes to the emergency room, the triage nurse or resident on call is likely to contact the therapist to ask what you would like done. Following the consultation-to-the-client strategy, you would first ask to speak with your client in order to discuss how going into the hospital does and does not coincide with the client's long-term goals and the agreed-upon treatment plan. You might then coach the client on how to communicate the plan to the ER staff and weigh in only if that is required for credibility. If the hospital staff were concerned about suicide risk and were reluctant to release the client, you would not advise the hospital staff to release the client but instead might coach the client on what he or she needed to do or say to appropriately address and thereby decrease the legitimate worries of the ER staff. In other words, your first move is consultation to the client, not environmental intervention.

Environmental Intervention

The DBT therapist does intervene in the environment on the client's behalf except, in some circumstances: when the short-term gain is worth the long-term loss in learning, when the client is unable to act on his or her own and outcome is very important, and when it is the humane thing to do and will cause no harm. In these cases, the therapist interacts with others in the client's life to provide information or serve as an advocate, or may directly enter the environment to give assistance. Even here the spirit is to strengthen the client's ability to advocate on his or her own behalf. You therefore dialectically balance environmental intervention and consultation to the patient. In meetings that you attend with the client, the client would primarily speak for him- or herself with you playing a supportive role. You would use your status to affirm the client's autonomy and capability.

Specific Dialectical Strategies

In addition to dialectically balancing problem solving and validation, reciprocal and irreverent communication, and consultation-to-the-patient with environmental intervention, several further specific dialectical strategies are also used to maintain movement. The therapist reaches for dialectical strategies when he or she is stuck. However, when we're stuck, we may feel frustrated or despairing and be prone to problematic use of dialectical strategies. Linehan gives a cautionary note in her treatment manual that I will paraphrase here because it is crucial: dialectical strategies can be easily confused with gimmicks and game playing. Therefore, the therapist needs to show the utmost care, honesty, and commitment to what is actually said and done, so that dialectical strategies are used with humility, and not from a superior position of "I know and am tricking you into seeing it my way."

Entering the Paradox

Clients face seemingly irresolvable dilemmas, including in therapy itself, which create impasse. For example, the therapist might suggest change on some problem behavior and the client might respond, "If you understood my suffering you wouldn't ask me to do something I can't do or that makes me feel worse than I already do." Rather than convince the client that things will eventually get better or that in fact she can do it, the therapist enters the paradox, but not in a rational way. Instead, the therapist highlights the paradoxical or contradictory elements without pulling the client out of the struggle and encourages the client to solve the dilemma experientially, to find how things can be true and not true, and that the answer can be both yes and no. Entering the paradox of needing the client to do more while in fact the client is doing all she can, the therapist might say, "I understand too well not to ask it. I can't think of anything more uncaring than to give up on you." Linehan (1993a) has highlighted common examples of these paradoxes in DBT. They include that the client is free to choose her own behavior but cannot stay in DBT if she does not choose to reduce intentional self-injury. The therapist genuinely cares for the client as a person, yet if the client stops paying for therapy, therapy stops. The therapist urges the client to get in control of her excessive urges to control. The therapist uses highly controlling techniques to increase the client's freedom.

Metaphor

Metaphors compare by analogy something the client understands to something he or she does not. A therapist can discuss difficult issues via metaphor without the client feeling controlled because points can be made indirectly. Because metaphors often have multiple meanings, the client can use it in his or her own way, feel more open, less overwhelmed, and less likely to stop listening. Many metaphors have already been used in this book, and common ones in DBT emphasize therapy as a journey or a climb the team makes together. Here's one example, used with clients: "It's hard to confidently lead the climb here when you keep unclipping the rope and jumping off the mountain." Two other examples position client difficulties as wholly understandable: being a rose in a tulip garden, climbing with an 80-pound pack while others on the path walk unburdened.

Devil's Advocate

In devil's advocate, the therapist holds down the maladaptive end of the continuum, freeing the client to advocate for the more adaptive end of the continuum. This technique is used to strengthen the client's position once he has moved toward adaptive responding. For example, after discussing the pros and cons of giving up suicidal behavior and beginning DBT, the client might tentatively say he wants to commit to a year of DBT. The therapist might then ask:

THERAPIST: Suicidal behavior has been your ace in the hole. Why would you want to enter a therapy where you have to give up suicide for a year?

CLIENT: I don't have a choice, this is the only real option.

THERAPIST: Yes, that's how it feels to me too, but you know, in the middle of the night, when things are hardest, you are going to want to say, "I give up. I can't do it." What you are signing on for right now, is that no matter how hard it gets, you won't do that, you'll take that option completely off the table for this year. Rather than throw in the towel, you'll use every new skill we work on and call me for help . . . that will really be hard. Personally, I think you will do great in this therapy, but the more important question is, are you really willing to go through those moments with suicide off the table?

Extending

Extending is used most often when the client attacks or communicates a threat. In extending, the therapist takes one aspect of the client's communication more seriously than the client anticipated, sometimes taking the client more seriously than she takes herself. The client, for example, may have been reinforced for making threats in past therapies and offer a threat or challenge when unhappy with the therapist's or program's limits. "If you don't act differently, this therapy isn't going to help me (the challenge)." To extend, the therapist might say, "If this therapy isn't helping, then we need to do something about that. Do you think you should fire me? This is very serious." Extending works best when the client is not expecting the therapist to take him or her seriously.

Activating Wise Mind

In DBT, the therapist assumes that the client has the capacity for wisdom, a way of knowing that integrates emotion and reason, grasping meaning or truth intuitively. In skills training, clients learn to deliberately cultivate this ability with various mindfulness techniques and guided imagery. The therapist may call on the client's wisdom when they reach a therapeutic impasse by asking, "What would wise mind say?" In a juvenile correctional facility once, a youth was getting wound up after a peer taunted him and then staff asked him to go to his room. As the emotion escalated, the youth's favorite staff called out to him, "Joe! What would wise mind say right now?" The youth completely shifted gears and said, "Go to my room and chill out, I want to go on the outing later." Even in the heat of a very intense moment, a client can often access the wisdom to know of what's needed.

Making Lemonade

In making lemonade out of lemons, the therapist helps the client transform something problematic into an asset. The therapist may view a discouraging event as an opportunity to practice distress tolerance. For example, a client had a male group leader who physically resembled the man who raped her and there were no other group openings. Therefore, the client and therapist made "lemonade out of lemons" in that they deliberately made contact with the make skills trainer during group as exposure therapy. At times, finding the good in difficult situations is like finding a needle in the haystack.

Allow Natural Change

The therapist does not artificially create stability and consistency. Instead, the therapist allows change to occur naturally to help the client develop comfort with change, ambiguity, unpredictability, and inconsistency, knowing that this too is an opportunity to practice acceptance of reality as it is. For example, say a very reliable and predictable therapist has a disruption at work and at home, and becomes less able to promptly return phone calls. This becomes an opportunity for the client to better gener-alize and independently use her skills to learn how caring can remain steady even when life circumstances mean delayed responses.

In moments when we're stuck, we may have habitual first moves such as to judge the other out of frustration or helplessness. From a dialectical perspective, the trick is to have a rapid second move to regain balance, such as to find and describe the web of causality where both the client's and your own responses are perfectly determined responses, and could not be otherwise. With practice, the sensations of being "stuck" with a client come to function as cues that prompt us to change our relationship to what is happening. We resume a dialectical stance that unites us in a nonresistive manner to what is actually happening. We remember we are connected and in this together (unity) rather than solely experiencing the rigid, dysregulated response, "I'm doing this to you; you are doing this to me" (duality). We remember that at any point, an opposite or complemen-tary point can be held that also has some validity. Dialectical strategies allow the therapist and client to move with contradictions and tensions toward reconciliation and resolution at increasingly functional and viable levels.

Dialectical thinking and strategies are most apparent and needed when there is conflict. The following extended example shows multiple points of conflict and dialectical strategies in action.

CASE EXAMPLE: YVETTE

Yvette is a 26-year-old who has made repeated suicide attempts beginning in her late teens. She had intense conflict with her parents. At her stepfa-ther's insistence, Yvette at 16 was sent to live in the country with a rela-tive to get her away from her "bad friends." She ran away back to the city and was raped while living on the streets. She became addicted to heroin, then slipped into prostitution to pay for drugs, and only managed to get out of it due to incredibly loyal friends. She kept all this secret from her parents but blamed them. She moved back in with her parents, resumed high school, and began cutting her arms with a razor to release the ten-sion. She made two suicide attempts, one at 17 and another at 19. Both attempts were followed by extended psychiatric hospitalizations, during which Yvette's suicidal behavior became more frequent and more medi-cally serious as a function of power struggles with staff. After the last discharge, she made good for a while. Her parents financed all expenses so she could complete her GED and then get an AA degree to do childcare work. She had nearly finished her degree when a chance meeting with an old boyfriend spiraled into a spontaneous trip to Mexico with him. He abandoned her there after an argument, stealing her purse and passport. By the time she sorted it all out and got home, she had missed final exams. She went to the school counselor and managed to negotiate "incompletes" with key professors. Again, her family knew nothing about this. She came home for winter break. One night she went out with friends, and when she came home drunk, violently argued with her stepfather. She took what would have been a lethal overdose but then got scared and drove to an emergency room. After a 72-hour hold, she went to a step-down day treatment program and then entered an outpatient DBT program.

In addition to the standard DBT goals, Yvette's personal goals included getting a full-time job and a better relationship with her mother. Yvette and her stepfather were estranged. On the advice of the parents' marital therapist, since the fight the stepfather refused to help Yvette financially, except to pay therapy and tuition bills, if and only if Yvette documented attendance and satisfactory progress. Three months into therapy, Yvette had reestablished some contact with her mother. She had part-time work as a waitress in a bar and was completing the remaining course work for her degree. However, Yvette was struggling. At the bar, Yvette received constant unwanted attention to her body. The late-night shift disrupted her sleep pattern. She found it increasingly difficult to concentrate while doing schoolwork. Schoolwork itself was more difficult to return to than she expected, and her perfectionism, combined with depressed mood and lowered functioning, created tremendous stress. As Yvette hit the end-of-semester crunch, her mother invited Yvette to attend her stepfather's retirement party. This invitation to an important family event was a major peace offering from her stepfather.

Yvette prepared thoroughly with her therapist about how to cope with the shame she anticipated feeling during the extended Saturday evening of contact with her family. Yvette followed the plan by taking brief breaks in the kitchen to regroup. Unexpectedly, the woman hired to cater the party spoke Spanish and Yvette enjoyed practicing her Spanish as a distraction. However, when Yvette stepped back into the dining room, a guest mistook her for a server, treating her in a highly condescending manner. Rather than correct his misperception, Yvette acted the subservient part, then laughed to herself as she walked back into the kitchen. Unbeknown to Yvette, her stepfather heard the entire interaction. He followed her into the kitchen and said, "That was unnecessary. Don't come here and humiliate me." Yvette handled it skillfully. She calmed her stepfather and apologized profusely, so that from her stepfather's point of view the air was cleared. Yvette then left early without saying goodbye. Her mother, noticing her absence later in the evening, heard the stepfather's version of events, and became concerned. When Yvette failed to answer her phone, her mother panicked and called Yvette's therapist. The therapist received the page, reached Yvette, and assessed suicide risk. Although suicide and self-harm urges were up, Yvette denied any plan. The therapist coached Yvette to text-message her mom ("Am safe & fine; sorry to worry you; didn't want to ruin Bill's party. At concert, can't talk, will call tomorrow."). Yvette also agreed to talk the next day with the therapist. The therapist called the mother to make sure she'd received the text message and to reassure her that Yvette was working hard in therapy.

Yvette called the therapist on Sunday, used coaching well, and felt the plan they had devised would get her through until the scheduled session on Tuesday. However, late Sunday night Yvette left a message on the therapist's work phone, speaking in a barely audible voice: "I can't do it. I'm hearing voices again . . . you are going to get burned out on me . . . I can't take it. . . . " The therapist heard the message on Monday morning, again spoke with Yvette and learned that she had spent Sunday night writing a good-bye letter to her mother. Despite Yvette's extreme passivity on the phone, the therapist managed to get Yvette to make an emergency appointment with her psychiatrist to get help with the psychotic symptoms and sleep.

On Monday afternoon, the therapist met with her DBT team and described her dilemmas: the client's apparent competence and history of being secretive made it hard to assess her suicide risk confidently; the options for reducing stressors, like withdrawing from school, would feel like a defeat to Yvette; and hospitalization had typically increased her suicidal behavior. On top of it all, the therapist had plans to go out of town the following weekend for the first time with a new boyfriend. A different teammate said, "For some reason I keep having this image of a horse caught in barbed wire. The more Yvette struggles, the more trapped she's getting and she's starting to switch between flailing and laying there passive because she knows she can't get out on her own." Another teammate chimed in, "Yeah, and you're urgent about cutting her out of there because your new cowboy might ride off into the sunset without you if you fart around too long with that damn horse!" The humor and metaphor helped the therapist settle down and reconnect with the need to go slow, to ask her client to "be still" and not do anything to make the situation worse, while they cut away the problems, strand by strand. The therapist also realized she needed to discuss whether she would take calls on her weekend away with her boyfriend. She wanted to be clear about her limits before she met with her client the next day.

The therapist left the meeting clear about her targets. Because she had so many targets and because Yvette was working hard, she decided to schedule a longer session in advance of the weekend and a coaching call on Saturday, in addition to arranging for Yvette's favorite skills trainer to be available on call for the weekend. In the time she had, the therapist needed to shift Yvette to a more active problem-solving stance so that they could avert hospitalization and a worsening of crisis. At a minimum, she needed to:

- Gain good information about suicide risk, knowing that apparent competence would require being persistent
- Treat the major problems that made suicide ideation spike to the point of writing a good-bye letter, namely:
  o Sleep disturbance and psychotic symptoms
  o Anticipation of failing school and facing humiliation from her stepfather.

In such crisis sessions, it is easy for therapists to bog down in power struggles by pushing too much for change and thereby evoking client resistance or by treating the client as overly fragile and thereby missing the opportunity to encourage use of new, more skillful behaviors in a crisis. A dialectical stance and dialectical balancing of strategies become essential.

The therapist began the session balancing stylistic communication strategies as she oriented Yvette to the need to take an active stance in the session. The therapist started in a reciprocal style, very warm and intense.

"Yvette, we're in a crisis here, right? And you worked great with me over the weekend, but I can feel you are slipping. I don't think you usually let people know that you are slipping so this is real progress. You and I were working great (*then slightly cooler and more matter-of-fact*) and then somehow Sunday night you went back to the old suicidal way of coping, writing a good-bye letter. . . . (*Then lightly, with a smile, irreverent.*) Not the new and improved response we're looking for. I think we should see if we can understand what made the suicide urges spike like that and then figure out how to get you through this without old behaviors. Even in the session today, let's see if I can help so you don't sink down into that old passivity. That seem good?"

As the therapist assessed what caused the suicidal ideation to spike, Yvette started talking in a blasé, singsong voice, fantasizing aloud.

"They really would be better off if I was dead. They wouldn't have to pay so much money for me, they wouldn't have to deal with me. I could make it be a good story too, because I could overdose on heroin—that would get them totally off the hook. Their friends would be *so* sympathetic. (*Then, in a slightly overdramatic voice.*): 'It's so sad! After all they did for that girl!' I wrote a great note."

The therapist views this as "old behavior" and takes a confrontational tone to help Yvette jump off of this unproductive track. Deadpan, the therapist says, "Shall I cue the dramatic music now? Maybe this is where the camera pans to your friends feeling like they failed you for the rest of their lives? *(irreverence)*." They both sit silently. The therapist then shifts forward in her chair (and again very intense but now quiet and warmly reciprocal), says, "Yvette, you are too close to the edge to pretend you don't matter. Let's get the pain down. Let's find our way through this together."

Yvette was able to identify that her urges to suicide would increase in the coming week when she felt she was failing at school. In particular, suicidal ideation would increase when she thought of the paper and exam due on the same day; she could not concentrate well enough to study and was struggling with auditory hallucinations. She believed her stepfather would pull the plug on funding school if she did poorly. At one point the therapist was pulling for Yvette to stay actively engaged in the conversation and to generate solutions despite feeling overwhelmed and hopeless. Yvette shouted at the therapist, "Don't you understand?! I can't do it!" The therapist had been focused on problem-solving change strategies but Yvette asserts her vulnerability. At this point, the therapist is tempted to shift focus and explore the possibility of Yvette withdrawing from college due to her understandable vulnerability. But that solution risks Yvette's further attack or withdrawal in the session because it would feel like the therapist does not believe in her; that her stepfather has been right all along; that there is nothing to live for because her "emotional problems" will always defeat her and life will be an unending series of failures.

Instead, the therapist responds dialectically by describing the typical pattern with empathy and validation, demonstrating she knows exactly where Yvette is located emotionally and in her pattern from past chain analyses before going back into problem solving.

> "Yvette, listen to me. Look at me. This is how it goes for you: things go well and then the stress really comes on and you white knuckle it or fantasize about killing yourself. No one around you has the slightest clue about how bad things are. Am I right? [Yvette nods.] This time you are doing it different, a way that could work for you because I see you hanging on by a thread here. You took action to get some help with your brain so it can sleep and get less psychotic. That's really good. That strengthens the thread you're holding. You've got me, we're a good team, and I know how bad off you are. That's good.

But you are getting tired. When you get tired, your mind resorts to suicide as a solution. Right about now, the old pattern is you quit, and kind of passively go down the tubes. I don't know how many times you can do that, survive that. You hate yourself for that. You start acting more and more out of control. Your parents move in to control you. You hate that. So we have a choice, OK? Either *you* are going to be in control here or someone else is. I vote for you. So, the problem we need to solve is what is better for you—is it better to withdraw on a medical leave, or is it better to talk with your professors and work out a way to finish. The skill here is pros and cons, you willing?—does this seem right for you?"

A short time later in the session, Yvette slipped into an angry tirade about how humiliating it was for her stepfather to require a weekly report. She was furious that her mother panicked and assumed the worst. The therapist responds irreverently.

"I believe we have barked up that tree before. This tree is where you want to scream 'YOU ARE SO UNREASONABLE!!!' (*playfully flailing both fists in a hilarious manner that makes Yvette laugh*). If you stand there yelling like a crazy woman, they will move in to control you and feel more distrusting of everything you say. You are scary when you act crazy, and they act crazy when you act crazy. That is not the tree we want. We want a new tree. The Yvette-is-handling-this-so-well tree, where they have to take you seriously and feel no need to control you. You are totally in control of how controlling they are."

With this last final comment, the therapist dialectically enters the paradox in the client's dilemma about control.

At another point, the therapist was helping Yvette generate ways to have more support. Yvette began to minimize this need and said she was pretty sure school and a weekend of unstructured time would work out. The therapist said, "You're like that Far Side cartoon where the guys in the lab coats have an impossible equation on the chalkboard and right in the middle it says, 'And then a miracle happens.'" Yvette smiled.

YVETTE: I wish a miracle *would* happen.

THERAPIST: I wonder what it would look like if it did—if you had the support you need?

YVETTE: I'd be able to go into a hospital but get out to do school and work, but I wouldn't be alone.

Yvette shuts down as she feels a wave of shame at how desperate she feels at needing help. The therapist doesn't have a lot of time left so instead of coaching Yvette to get the shame down, goes for humor to help Yvette regulate shame.

THERAPIST: You know Annie LaMott? She says, "My mind is a like a bad neighborhood. I try never to go there alone." That definitely is the motto we need right now. Where can we get you more support?

YVETTE: I don't know.

THERAPIST: Well, what would wise mind say?

YVETTE: I don't know.

THERAPIST: Let's just check, OK? (*Leads a wise-mind exercise of asking the question and listening for the answer.*)

YVETTE: (*After several minutes, very calmly.*) . . . I should stay with Diane, she can be my hospital. I'll make a schedule, just like I would if I went to St. Mark's. Frozen dinners.

THERAPIST: OK. How's that feel?

YVETTE: I hadn't even thought of her. She'd do it.

THERAPIST: Got her number?

YVETTE: Yes.

THERAPIST: Let's call her now.

In the end, the therapist and client devised a crisis plan. Yvette wrote a note to her parents, explaining the increase in psychotic symptoms and ways that made school more difficult and asking their advice. She stayed with a friend for 24/7 support. She negotiated out of one school assignment so she could focus exclusively on the other. She took an extra weekend waitress shift to stay active rather than ruminate. The therapist's clarity about her availability pushed them to develop a more adequate plan and, knowing her therapist was stretching to do a call one day during her weekend, touched and motivated Yvette. As she relied more on the therapist, she acted more skillfully; this then meant that her parents relaxed and were less coercive.

The key dialectic of change in the context of accepting present reality often takes the form of combining polar opposites in the same breath—the therapeutic "Yes, and": "You are doing the very best you can and you need to try harder." The ratio of validation to problem solving shifts, depending on the circumstances. Balance might come from emphasizing change or acceptance over time. Or the therapist may need to move rapidly from position to position so that the client is off balance and kept from locking down into a rigid position. It's the ability to make rapid shifts in order to keep balanced movement that is essential. The dialectical stance and specific strategies described in this chapter are meant to help the therapist move with whole hearted certainty, strength, and total commitment yet exquisite sensitivity to the balance of acceptance and change that leads to forward movement. The next chapter shows how the therapist integrates the change, acceptance, and dialectical strategies discussed so far to get the most movement in each clinical interaction.

SIX

Assess, Motivate, and Move

Getting the Most from Each Interaction

Now that Chapters 3, 4, and 5 have detailed use of the core strategies, I return in this chapter to DBT's framework for clinical decision making introduced in Chapter 2. In that chapter I explained how the therapist arrives at an initial case formulation by identifying likely controlling variables for primary target behaviors. In this chapter, I describe how sessions unfold after the pretreatment period with attention to how the therapist decides, moment to moment, what to treat and how.

Actively formulating the client's problems, planning treatment, and intervening continues in each clinical interaction, and there are multiple interactions over the course of a session. When you are finding your way through difficult terrain, you must first get the lay of the land. That is, at the beginning of each clinical contact, you assess to get a general sense of where you and the client are and how that relates to where you and the client want to go. Then you motivate. Make sure your client agrees and is willing to go the route you propose under his or her own power, rather than being dragged along. Finally, you move—you intervene to create as much movement toward the client's goals as you can. These broad steps appear straightforward but, with "wicked problems," there are so many complicated relationships and dependencies that it's easy to lose the forest for the trees. Therefore, I've broken these steps down into five key tasks and organized them into the decision tree shown in Figure 6.1.

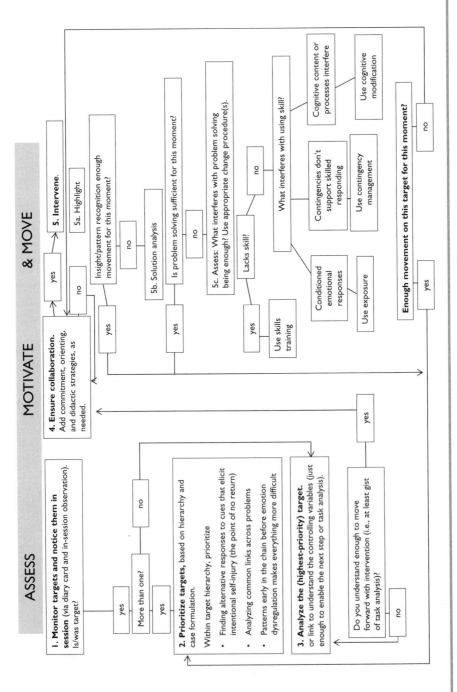

FIGURE 6.1. Assess, motivate, and move: Steps in using behavioral assessment and intervention.

ASSESS: LOCATE WHERE WE ARE

Task 1: Monitor Targets and Notice Them in Session

At the beginning of an interaction, locate where the client is with respect to problems and progress. You do this by reviewing the client's diary card, listening to the client's report of her week, and directly observing the client in session. As explained in Chapter 3, the standard DBT diary card (see Figure 3.1) helps the therapist quickly see what clinically relevant behavior is on the scene (see also Figure 3.3). Each day the client monitors all primary treatment targets and records information on the diary card. You can add weekly or periodic standardized measures or measures specifically tailored to the individual as needed. The client brings the completed diary card to each session and typically, sessions begin with the two of you reviewing the diary card together.

Expect the very problems that occur in the person's life to interfere with completing the diary card. For example, if the client struggles with intense shame about his behavior, the client may avoid noting problems on the diary card in order to avoid increased feelings of shame. If the client is couch surfing between friends' apartments, she may not be able to locate her diary card amid the chaos of her living situation. In either case, the diary card itself becomes an opportunity to work on common links across problems in the client's life. So, for example, when a client forgets to bring in her diary card, do a brief chain analysis of what interfered: did she in fact leave the last session committed to doing it? Did she remember it during the week? If she intended and remembered, what interfered with completing the diary card? Often the links that lead to an incomplete or forgotten diary card are the same as those that lead to other problems.

As you scan the diary card together, look for instances of progress or problems and for patterns. Wonder aloud with the client about functional relationships among behaviors reported on the card. For example, "I see that on these two days where you drank less, fear and shame were much higher—did you notice that? Are those related?"

In addition to the diary card, you are directly observing the client and the client is telling you what was important about the week. The second job, then, is to notice when clinically relevant behaviors (either problems or progress) are occurring in the session (Tsai et al., 2008). Whenever you notice them, from reports about daily life between sessions or in session, you use the opportunity to strengthen progress and facilitate needed changes. This can often be done briefly with a validating comment or through highlighting.

Task 2: Prioritize Targets—What Must Get Attention

Often more than one target behavior has happened during the week or is happening in session. When several targets need therapeutic attention, use the target hierarchy and case formulation *together* to determine the priority of treatment tasks. Let's work through an example to illustrate how to use both to decide among priorities.

Since the last session, Karrie burned herself with a cigarette, and left a voicemail, sounding drugged, murmuring so quietly that the therapist could not make out what she said. In addition, you now learn that Karrie also faces two situations in the coming week that could easily become crises: she will lose her housing if she mishandles a conversation with her roommate and she is interviewing for a new job. If you had 50 minutes with her, how would you allocate them?

Applying the Stage 1 target hierarchy, you would prioritize whatever is needed to decrease the probability of life-threatening behaviors such as intentional self-injury (Target 1). Then, you would prevent or resolve problems in the therapy relationship itself (Target 2). Then you would help Karrie with severe quality-of-life issues (Target 3) and with applying the skills needed to support all of the above (Target 4). In an optimal session, you would try to get as much movement on as many targets as possible. Using only the target hierarchy to prioritize session time gives the following working agenda of the therapy tasks to accomplish:

1. Prevent future self-injury. Do chain analysis to understand the variables that led Karrie to burn herself along with solution analysis to identify how Karrie can handle a similar context differently next time; check what happened with commitment to stop self-injury and revisit commitment as needed.
2. Decrease therapy-interfering behavior. Do what's needed to decrease the probability of another problematic phone message— most likely, chain analysis, solution analysis, and perhaps contingency clarification and management will be used.
3. Decrease quality-of-life interfering behaviors. Help with issues of roommate and job interview if there's time.

However, the target hierarchy is not a set of rules; it is a set of *guidelines* to be used in tandem with the case formulation. For this particular client, losing her housing or handling the job interview poorly will mean she must ask her parents for money. Asking for money will prompt Karrie to feel humiliated and prompt her parents to be harshly critical of her— the very circumstances associated with her past suicide attempts. The formulation suggests that if you fail to treat the quality-of-life issues, the probability of a suicide attempt will increase (Target 1). In this case, the best way to treat Target 1 is to help Karrie prepare to be successful with the roommate and the job interview. These therapy tasks would trump other agenda items because they influence the probability of imminent suicide crisis behavior. Decreasing the risk of suicide completion is a higher priority than the intentional self-injury of burning.

This example shows why analyzing the function of behavior is so important. To identify the highest-priority target requires you to understand the pattern of controlling variables. It would be a mistake to focus on the form (e.g., "This is quality-of-life-interfering, therefore lower priority"). It is better to focus on the function ("This quality-of-life issue is functionally related to suicide attempts"). If instead, conflict with the therapist was associated with past increases in suicidal behavior, then failing to address the client's problematic phone message might precipitate a suicidal crisis. If that were true, then the top priority would be resolving the therapy-interfering behavior of therapist and client regarding phone messages because working on that would most directly decrease the probability of suicide crisis behaviors. The target hierarchy should always be used in conjunction with the case formulation, rather than used in a rule-bound or unsophisticated way.

To "locate" the client, you look at the current circumstances and quite literally work to determine if the client is on the path to a target behavior. For one client, you might realize she is en route to self-harm as soon as you see the two variables most associated with past incidents of serious self-harm: she is dissociating in session and she is heading into an unstructured weekend. Knowing the client and reading the terrain you prioritize treating dissociation to reduce the risk of intentional self-injury. For a second client, however, dissociating often leads her to sleep away the hours—dissociating moves her *off* the path to intentional self-injury (but perhaps onto the path of being fired for missing work). Knowing the particular chain and path along which the client's behavior tends to travel determines how you prioritize treatment tasks. If Karrie is en route to a suicide crisis, how far exactly is she along that path—near to it, far from it, moving slowly or moving fast? Where are alternate paths that she could take to move her toward her goals yet avoid suicidal behavior?

Prioritizing therapy tasks by using the target hierarchy in the context of the formulation gives you an idea of what you hope to accomplish in the session. As you learn more during your conversation, priorities may shift or become clearer. This leads us to the next step.

Task 3: Analyze the Highest-Priority Target—
Where Are the Forks in the Road?

Once you have an overview of the client's clinically relevant target behaviors and how to prioritize them, the next task is to assess specific instances of the highest priority target. Use chain analysis until you have a clear enough sense of controlling variables to allow intervention. Chain analysis begins with explicit or implicit client consent to the question, "Can we look closely at this together?" Make sure the client is willing to collaborate on the task. If you detect reluctance, shift to motivating the client (see Task 4), and come back to the chain analysis.

Often it makes the most sense to work on two places in chain analysis first. One is the point of no return, the place in the sequence where you want the client, no matter what, to have the ability to step back and not engage in the problem behavior. The second place is early in the sequence before emotion dysregulation makes it difficult to change course. This is often close to the first cues on the path to the problem behavior.

MOTIVATE

Task 4: Ensure Collaboration

Any time you assess or move for change, make sure you have (and keep) sufficient collaboration to do the work. The client should begin any therapy task well oriented. She should see vividly why a behavior is problematic with respect to her goals and how making a change would move her toward her goals. It is as if, prior to initiating change, you pull out the map and say to the client, "You are here. We want to go here, correct? See how continuing with this current behavior takes you off track? An alternative route is needed to get from where you are to where you want to go. Wouldn't you agree?"

Constantly monitor whether the client agrees enough to work well with you on the therapy task. This need not be elaborate or explicit: sometimes the implicit agreement is so clear that therapy is two well-matched horses harnessed to the same task. At other times, the therapist may assume agreement, but has lost the client. The client may subtly balk for any number of reasons. When you detect the client's reluctance, shift to whatever work is needed by you or the client to regain collaboration. For example, sometimes a client does not understand how what you propose is relevant, or the client has the sense that you do not truly understand the problem. In this case, you must shift to assessment to gain a more accurate understanding of the client's point of view, or to didactic or orienting strategies to convey that you do have an accurate understanding.

At other times, the client understands the therapy task and its rationale but is ambivalent. Here, commitment itself becomes an explicit focus of work. You do what is needed, whenever needed, to maintain genuine collaboration.

Concretely, then, any change intervention (including chain analysis) begins with explicit or implicit consent to the question, "Can we work on this in the following way?" Depending on what is needed in the moment, the therapist may articulate the problem and therapy task in a manner that self-evidently connects with the client's current state, or the therapist may boldly step into the heart of the matter with a nonjudgmental but confrontive stance. The guidelines described in the chapters on validation and dialectics (Chapters 4 and 5, respectively) then come into play. For example, the therapist may need to fully and vividly validate the client's reservations, oscillating between a warm, reciprocal style and an irreverent style while using the freedom-to-choose, absence-of-alternatives commitment strategy to strengthen collaboration.

MOVE TOWARD THE CLIENT'S GOALS

Once you have a general sense of the priority of needed therapy tasks and of the client's motivation, then collaborative work on the highest-priority tasks begins. "Work" can take many forms and needn't be defined only as use of a change-oriented strategy. Assessment alone may be sufficient work, particularly if it serves as exposure therapy or focuses on observing and describing emotion to strengthen adaptive responding. Creating even a millimeter of change may be sufficient work in a given moment. The focus of work may shift as assessment shows you other dysfunctional links, or as other dysfunctional links occur in session. Whenever there is a "workable moment," you work there until there is some change, movement, or strengthening of clinical progress or until some higher priority target trumps it. By workable moment, I mean your and the client's sense that some movement is possible in the time available, given all the other important tasks on the docket and the client's capability in the moment.

When you discern an important link, particularly if you think it goes across problems, you may reshuffle the priority of therapy tasks to give you time to address that link. For example, you might notice on the diary card that the client consumed five beers and had a spike of urges to self-harm on Friday night. As you begin to do a chain analysis together, you learn your client loaned her car to a friend who drinks heavily. In an instant, the deck of therapy tasks may need to be reshuffled. You would rapidly consider your case formulation, especially remembering the probable controlling variables for highest-priority targets. If this is the beginning of a repeating pattern of crisis-generating behavior, she doesn't get her car back as planned and misses work when she's already on the brink of being fired or if she ends up in a huge argument as happened last time about him being irresponsible—would either of these events increase the risk of a suicidal crisis? If so, the conversation might pivot to head off a crisis while she is still early in the sequence; make sure she has a fool proof plan to cope with the worst-case scenarios without resorting to suicidal behavior. If neither event would increase risk of suicidal behavior, then you might simply highlight the repeated pattern of making problematic choices with this guy and agree in the near future to assess what can be done to decrease crisis-generating behaviors.

You get what you can take; you take what you can get. The therapist, at any given moment, knows the therapy tasks on the table and works on the one that fits the moment, that is, balances what's most important with the client's capability and the time available. With a client who is extremely sensitive to negative feedback, there may be no way to bring up her therapy-interfering behavior unless you have most of a session available to help her regulate enough to let in the feedback and make sure she leaves the session in good shape. A different client, who can take a full body blow of criticism, might laugh you off with something like "People always tell me that. I'll work on it." When the client is in the midst of crises, you have only a brief time, like a boxing coach or a corner man between rounds. You must rapidly address the highest priority to get the boxer back into shape to continue the fight.

Task 5: Intervene

When you see forks in the road where the client might do something differently and thereby make progress, then intervene with highlighting, solution analysis, or one or more of the four change procedures (skills training, exposure, contingency management, and cognitive modification; see Figure 6.1). In other words, you recall your basic task analysis of how to replace old behavior with new behavior. You have three basic choices of how intensively you will intervene based on how the case formulation and exact moment match up.

Option 5a: Highlighting

To highlight, briefly comment on a specific instance of the client's behavior and its implications, saying things like, "Have you noticed that . . . ?" or "Don't you think it's interesting that . . . ?" Highlighting comments alone can prompt change. For example, a therapist playfully said to his client, "Have you noticed you start every reasonable request with, 'I'm sorry to bother you?' That's kind of interesting, don't you think?" and the client replied, "I should knock that off, huh? It's me going with the action urge of guilt like we talked about at skills training." From then on, the client began to self-correct the overly apologetic style. Highlighting comments are also used to point out dysfunctional behavior when you don't have enough time to really work on it but you don't want to let it slip by without comment.

Option 5b: Solution Analysis

When more than highlighting is needed, solution analysis might be the best way forward. This can take the form of a minimal intervention, such as the therapist suggesting a solution that the client hadn't considered. At other times, an extended solution analysis is required as shown in Chapter 3 with Michael's sleep problem. This consists of identifying the problem, brainstorming solutions, selecting a solution, implementing the solution, and then evaluating its outcome with careful attention to troubleshooting and generalization. You combine many core strategies as you conduct solution analysis to ensure the client stays sufficiently motivated and committed to doing the work.

Option 5c: Skills Training, Exposure, Contingency Management, and Cognitive Modification Procedures

When analyzing the problem, suggesting solutions, orienting to treatment, giving information, and getting a commitment (i.e., mostly just talking) do not work, you return to basic behavior therapy assessment questions. You ask: Does the client have the skill required for this to go differently? If not, then use skills training procedures. If the client has the skill yet is not acting skillfully, then what gets in the way: Emotional reactions? Contingencies? Cognitive processes or content? Sometimes you must do a fair amount of work using one of the four change procedures to establish more adaptive behavior.

Decide how in depth to intervene based on how the case formulation fits the moment you are in. Keep the target hierarchy in mind. It's more important to prevent future serious problem behavior than to analyze the past, so prioritize work that will decrease the probability of the client taking the path toward high-priority targets. It's often smart to work at the point of no return so the client has a way to get through the very worst circumstance without life-threatening behaviors. It is often easiest to work earlier in the sequence of events that led to extreme behavior because at that point the client is still emotionally regulated. It's more efficient to work common links across chains.

CASE EXAMPLE: KARRIE

Let's now return to the example of Karrie to illustrate the decision making I've been describing. I'll start over from the beginning and go through the course of a single session. As we saw earlier, the therapist knows several priority targets before the session starts. To recap, Karrie burned herself with a cigarette since the last session and left a mumbled phone message. In the coming week, she has a job interview and she could lose her housing if she mishandles a conversation with her roommate. If either goes wrong, she will need to ask her parents for money. The hard criticism from her parents and subsequent humiliation are associated with past suicide attempts. Therefore, Karrie's case formulation suggests that these quality-of-life issues are functionally related to increased suicide risk and therefore likely to become the highest treatment priority for this session.

Task 1: Monitor Targets and Notice Them in Session

The therapist's first therapy task is to clarify the working agenda for the session. She needs to locate where she and the client are and prioritize where to work. When the therapist meets Karrie in the waiting area for her appointment, Karrie looks and talks as if she is in a high-emotion state.

Remember that using the three priority targets discussed above, our tentative agenda going into the session so far is to (1) decrease the probability of suicidal behavior and most likely the best way to do this will be to help her be successful with her roommate and the job interview and thereby avoid the highly critical triggering interactions she has with her parents if she fails; (2) prevent future nonsuicidal self-injury of burning herself; (3) do what's needed to decrease problematic phone messages.

As they sit down, Karrie hands the therapist her diary card (see Figure 6.2). Karrie often forgets her diary card and therefore, a first little therapy task is to strengthen this improvement. The therapist had carefully assessed, rather than assumed, whether the consequences she provided actually reinforced the desired behavior (contingency management). Comments like "great job on your diary card" were aversive to Karrie; such comments set off shame that she didn't do the card more regularly in the past and so inadvertently punished the behavior. Instead, small comments were much more reinforcing, such as, "It is so helpful to see how things have been for you." The therapist has gradually used these to shape better compliance with the diary card.

Dialectical Behavior Therapy **Diary Card**	Instructions: Circle the days you worked on each skill		Filled out in session? Y (N)		How often did you fill out this side? ___ Daily _X_ 2–3x ___ Once		
1. Wise mind	(Mon)	Tues	Wed	Thurs	Fri	Sat	Sun
2. Observe: just notice (Urge Surfing)	(Mon)	Tues	Wed	Thurs	Fri	Sat	Sun
3. Describe: put words on	Mon	Tues	Wed	Thurs	Fri	Sat	Sun
4. Participate: enter into the experience	Mon	Tues	Wed	Thurs	Fri	Sat	Sun
5. Nonjudgmental stance	(Mon)	Tues	Wed	Thurs	Fri	Sat	Sun
6. One-mindfully: in-the-moment	Mon	(Tues)	Wed	Thurs	Fri	Sat	Sun
7. Effectiveness: focus on what works	Mon	Tues	Wed	Thurs	Fri	Sat	Sun
8. Objective effectiveness: DEAR MAN	Mon	Tues	Wed	Thurs	Fri	Sat	Sun
9. Relationship effectiveness: GIVE	Mon	Tues	Wed	Thurs	Fri	Sat	Sun
10. Self-respect effectiveness: FAST	Mon	Tues	Wed	Thurs	Fri	Sat	Sun
11. Reduce vulnerability: PLEASE	(Mon	Tues	Wed)	Thurs	Fri	Sat	Sun
12. Build MASTERY	Mon	Tues	Wed	Thurs	Fri	Sat	Sun
13. Build positive experiences	Mon	Tues	Wed	Thurs	Fri	Sat	Sun
14. Opposite-to-emotion action (Alt. Rebellion)	Mon	(Tues)	Wed	Thurs	Fri	Sat	Sun
15. Distract (Adaptive Denial)	Mon	Tues	Wed	Thurs	Fri	Sat	Sun
16. Self-soothe	(Mon	Tues)	Wed	Thurs	Fri	Sat	Sun
17. Improve the moment	Mon	Tues	Wed	Thurs	Fri	Sat	Sun
18. Pros and cons	(Mon	Tues)	Wed	Thurs	Fri	Sat	Sun
19. Radical Acceptance	Mon	Tues	Wed	Thurs	Fri	Sat	Sun
20. Building Structure // Work	(Mon	Tues)	Wed	Thurs	Fri	Sat	Sun
21. Building Structure // Love	Mon	Tues	Wed	Thurs	Fri	Sat	Sun
22. Building Structure // Time	Mon	Tues	Wed	Thurs	Fri	Sat	Sun
23. Building Structure // Place	Mon	Tues	Wed	Thurs	Fri	Sat	Sun

Urge to use (0–5):	Before therapy session: 4	After therapy session: ___	
Urge to quit therapy (0–5):	Before therapy session: 2	After therapy session: ___	BRTC Card
Urge to suicide (0–5):	Before therapy session: 3	After therapy session: ___	

Dialectical Behavior Therapy **Diary Card**	Initials KS	ID#	Filled out in session (Y) N	How often did you fill out this side? ___ Daily _X_ 2–3x ___ Once	Date started

Some columns

Day & Date	URGES TO...			EMOTIONS					DRUGS								ACTIONS				
	Use	Suicide	S-H	Phys. Pain	Sad Grief	Shame	Anger Irr.	Fear Anx.	Illicit Drugs		ETOH	Prescription		OTC		S-H	Lying	Joy	Skills	R
	0–5	0–5	0–5	0–5	0–5	0–5	0–5	0–5	# Specify		# Specify	# Specify		# Specify		Y/N	#	0–5	0–5	✓
Mon	2	1	1	0	0	2	2	2								N	0		5	
Tues	2	2	2	0	2	2	0	2								N	0		4	
Wed	2	1	2	0	2	2	0	2								N	0		5	
Thur	2	2	2	2	2	2	4	4								N	0			
Fri	2	3	5	2	4	4	4	4								N	0			
Sat	2	4	2	4	4	4	4	4								Y	0			
Sun	2	5	1	2	4	5	5	5								N	0			

Apparently Unimportant Behaviors: Keeping Doors to Use Open:	*USED SKILLS 0 = Not thought about or used 1 = Thought about, not used, didn't want to 2 = Thought about, not used, wanted to 3 = Tried but couldn't use them	4 = Tried, could do them but they didn't help 5 = Tried, could use them, helped 6 = Didn't try, used them, didn't help 7 = Didn't try, used them, helped

FIGURE 6.2. Karrie's diary card.

As the therapist looks at the diary card, she can see that Karrie left multiple columns blank and she can't interpret blanks. So one task is to get this information. She needs to do this quickly, however, because she has multiple high-priority tasks. Therefore, as the session begins, the therapist might talk through the diary card with Karrie like this:

> "Let's take a look together at your diary card. (*Turns her chair so both can see it.*) Wow, Karrie, what a hard week, even at a glance. Man, one thing about these diary cards is it gives me immediate empathy. (*Says this as she looks up from the card, kindly but briefly making eye contact with Karrie. Then continues matter-of-factly with her gaze back on the diary card; Level 3 validation and likely reinforcement of completing diary card.*)
>
> "Let's see . . . OK. (*Highlighting.*) I can't see what's up when these columns for over-the-counter meds and alcohol are left blank." (*Highlighting.*)

Karrie responds that she had one beer, so little an amount that she didn't think to record it; she never uses over the counter medications except occasional ibuprofen. Spontaneously, she takes the card back and fills in the blanks, as she talks. Handing it back to the therapist, the therapist comments, "That works great, I see."

In the above exchange, the therapist has attempted to reinforce progress on filling out the diary card through low-key warmth and then uses highlighting to shape further use of the diary card. Highlighting was all that was needed and is likely to decrease the probability of incorrectly filled out diary cards the next time. The therapist continues:

THERAPIST: The first thing that really stands out is the Y in the self-harm column, that's what you mentioned in your message, right, about burning your arm? (*Since the last session, Karrie has burnt her arm with a cigarette and left a mumbled phone message for the therapist.*)

KARRIE: Yeah. (*Nods.*) I was pretty disappointed in myself. I haven't done anything since I started therapy.

THERAPIST: Yeah, I know, you've really been working hard. (*Tone is solemn, and she pauses, before resuming a more matter-of-fact pace.*) It's a big deal. I can see how disappointed you are. You really want to change, so we'll put that on our agenda and figure out what happened. (*Level 3 validation of Karrie's intent and Level 5 of her understandable disappointment with herself.*) But also, I'm just seeing this huge jump in suicidal ideation, from 1s and 2s to 5s [to higher-intensity ratings] and then you've got a lot of skills going on early in the week and then those drop off or what . . . ? Why the blanks here? (*Again, very matter-of-*

fact, nonjudgmental voice tone. The therapist rapidly oscillates stylistic strategies through the session thus far, sometimes warmer, sometimes cooler, dialectically balancing acceptance and change, to help Karrie stay regulated.)

KARRIE: Not sure—don't really remember why I didn't fill that out.

THERAPIST: Well, maybe as we go we can see if there were any places where skills might have helped, because this looks like you really needed more options . . . OK, so I'd say we spend most of our time today on helping you with whatever's got suicidal ideation going up so high and your urges to harm yourself up so high. Does that make sense? (*Checks collaboration.*)

KARRIE: Yes.

Task 2: Prioritize Targets

The therapist is figuring out priorities. She will need to ask assessment questions to find out whether Karrie is on the path toward a suicide crisis, as she suspects. If she learns Karrie is not on that path, then the therapist may need to choose between analyzing the conditions that led to the non-suicidal self-harm or the spike in suicidal ideation, depending on what poses the higher threat to the client's life. The therapist also would want to reestablish Karrie's commitment to stopping nonsuicidal self-injury. As they set the agenda in the last exchange above, the therapist assumes the best—that Karrie's disappointment reflects continued commitment to abstain from intentional self-injury as they'd agreed in pretreatment. But she wants to come back to assess if this assumption is correct. The other target behavior from the past week was the phone message. Untreated, this behavior will eventually burn out the therapist. The therapist rapidly decides that early in the session may be the only moment to do a little work on phone messages before she and the client become absorbed in work on the highest priorities. Therefore, the therapist switches gears to set up a brief chain analysis of the therapy-interfering behavior.

Task 3: Analyze Therapy-Interfering Phone Message

THERAPIST: One quick thing before we jump in: remember the phone message you left me last night? That was hard for me because you sounded almost drugged. What was going on with that, what made your speech so slurred? (*Steps in where angels fear to tread.*)

KARRIE: I took my sleeping pills but I still couldn't get my mind to stop, so I decided to call you but by then the medicine had kicked in and I was falling asleep.

THERAPIST: Would you be willing to call me *before* you take your medication so that I don't get worried? Or maybe I should be worried—did you take an overdose?

KARRIE: No, I just took the right dose.

Tasks 5a, 5c: Phone Message Intervention

THERAPIST: Good. OK. Once you're that groggy and out of it, be sure to tell me, "If I sound funny it's just that I took sleep medication, I did not OD." OK? Because it was really confusing.

KARRIE: Sure.

This small amount of highlighting and contingency clarification may be enough to decrease the probability of this therapy-interfering behavior occurring again. However, as Karrie says "Sure," the therapist notices a very slight change in Karrie's posture. Karrie shifts back, her eyes dart away, and her body crumples a tiny bit; she deflates as if she'd let a little air out of a balloon. The therapist wonders if Karrie feels shame and has started to hide a little or pull back due to the feedback about the phone call. If so, she needs to help Karrie stay emotionally regulated enough that she retains the capacity to do the highest-priority treatment tasks. The therapist again goes back to highlighting.

Tasks 1, 5a: In-Session Emotion Dysregulation

THERAPIST: Hey, did something just happen there? Did you just pull back a little?

KARRIE: (*Gives a tiny smile to acknowledge the therapist is on track.*)

THERAPIST: (*Asks gently and warmly.*) What would happen if you were to move in a little and not pull back because we've got a lot of things, obviously, from your diary card that are really troubling you. (*Connects task to client goals.*)

Here the therapist made a rapid decision not to work more explicitly for two reasons. First, they have the possibility of a suicide crisis on the horizon, so she wants to conserve time for that. Second, Karrie's sensitivity to shame means any direct targeting of it here will likely increase shame to the point that she is too dysregulated to work on anything else. Therefore, the therapist opts for a little highlighting in a reciprocal communication style and it works. Karrie shifts body posture and eye contact to engage.

Task 1: Assess Imminent Suicide Risk

They are now about 10 minutes into the session. The therapist and Karrie quickly assess imminent suicide risk. The therapist weaves risk assessment into review of the diary card. "So what was this '5' on suicidal ideation like for you on Sunday? Did you plan to kill yourself?" Karrie reassures the therapist that she had no plan and no intent, just ideation. But Karrie does say she worries about her ability to control herself if she doesn't get the job and things don't go well with the roommate this week.

This confirms that the problems with the job and the roommate are the main places Karrie and the therapist should work, but to be sure of priorities the therapist still needs to assess how dangerous the nonsuicidal self-injury was.

Task 3: Analyze Self-Harm Cigarette Burn: Where Are the Forks in the Road?

Task 4: Ensure Collaboration/Commitment

Task 5: Intervene

The therapist does a brief chain analysis (Task 3) and learns that Karrie relapsed after a friend left a cigarette lighter in her apartment. Karrie has already thrown out the lighter. Karrie works readily to generate and commit to a realistic one–two–three plan to immediately and skillfully prevent another relapse if she is inadvertently tempted when others put means in front of her (Task 5). From past experience, Karrie knows she should (1) remove the means or remove herself; (2) get support and accountability by calling a friend or the therapist and reasserting her commitment to never harm herself again and alert them she needs help; (3) if needed, go to the 24-hour café near her apartment with her skills manual and wait it out until she's 100% certain she won't self-harm. That plan and a quick strengthening of commitment (Task 4) is sufficient work to reduce the immediate probability of intentional self-injury by burning, even though it takes only 5 minutes.

Remember, you are going for "sufficient" movement. The priority of a target does not always directly equate with amount of session time. A high-priority target may only need 5 minutes when the therapist and client rapidly find their way and move forward as Karrie and her therapist do here. What's required is that you treat the highest-priority target sufficiently, not necessarily exclusively. The therapist must balance and realign priorities as the moment unfolds and new information is encountered.

Task 3: Analyze Spike in Suicidal Ideation: Where Are the Forks in the Road?

Now 20 minutes into the session, they begin a chain analysis to identify the controlling variables for the spike in suicidal ideation. Based on Karrie's last serious suicide attempt, the therapist hypothesizes that the most difficult thing for her may be the feeling of being trapped and humiliated if she must ask her parents for help. The therapist offers that idea to Karrie.

THERAPIST: Karrie, sometimes we've seen this kind of spike in suicidal ideation when you feel trapped and begin to feel humiliated that you might need financial help.

KARRIE: (*Immediately her emotions flare up.*) I'm not crawling to them for help! I can't do it—I'd rather be dead. I HATE THIS!

THERAPIST: (*Responds by orienting Karrie and then offering two options for therapy task, but as she does so she dramatically shifts her voice tone and body posture, leaning forward, lowering her volume yet speaking intensely, in a way that captures Karrie's attention, and communicates that she is taking Karrie's distress ultraseriously.*) Karrie, listen, suicidal ideation goes up when you face humiliation. Those are paired for you. As soon as you fear humiliation, your brain's solution is "suicide" to get you out of any chance of being humiliated. Does that fit? (*Checks on collaboration.*) Right now, me just saying the words, that it might happen, got your emotions up, right? You look panicky—like dread and shame are really firing even at the thought of asking your parents for help. (*Level 3 validation-articulating emotions that have not fully been expressed.*)

KARRIE: I'm not doing it!

THERAPIST: I'm fine with that. Listen, look at me for a sec, listen, all your emotions are firing, OK, can you tell? (*Micro-orients.*) Am I right, is it dread, and panic and . . . what do you feel?

KARRIE: My whole body is like NO! I want to scream.

THERAPIST: OK. So your whole body is responding to threat. Where's your suicide ideation now?

KARRIE: Off the chart, like 5+++.

THERAPIST: So your brain, as soon as it feels the threat of humiliation from your parents, goes to suicide as the way out. Have you noticed that? (*Highlights.*)

KARRIE: (*Nods.*)

THERAPIST: Are you tracking me here, or are you too much in emotion mind? Maybe say back to me what you are hearing me say so I can help tell how dysregulated you are. (*Karrie is tracking and shows she's got the gist of the pattern. With this degree of collaboration and orientation, the therapist then offers the therapy tasks.)*

Task 5c: In-Session Emotion Dysregulation, Skills Intervention

THERAPIST: You just did a great job—you had a big surge of emotion and now you're back with me, right? OK, what skill can you use right here to keep soothing your physiology? We need to be able to really work together. So what skill can you use now? *(Task 5c.)*

KARRIE: I brought a soda, let me get that out of my bag. Breathing works for me, really counting breaths.

Task 5b: Solution Analysis for Roommate Conversation and Job Interview

THERAPIST: Great.

KARRIE: *(Settles further with soda in hand and has taken several deep soothing breaths.)*

THERAPIST: *(Continues.)* What you just did is excellent; you're helping your physiology, super. Now, we need to help your brain have some other solutions. We need two things, OK? One: we have to decrease the threat of being humiliated. That means we'd work on the problems that are making you feel vulnerable, do whatever we can to work things out with your roommate and do a good interview. That make sense? *(checking collaboration)*

KARRIE: Yes.

THERAPIST: That's option 1—change the situation. Your body screams "No!" and you say, "OK, what is the threat? What can I do to avoid feeling humiliated?" Solve the problem, reduce the cue. You say it— put it in your own words so I know you're with me, OK?

KARRIE: *(Repeats, clearly showing she gets it.)*

THERAPIST: *(Stands and writes that potential therapy task using Karrie's words on the whiteboard, knowing this will further help Karrie remain regulated.)* Then option 2 is: we should help you regulate shame and humiliation. It's like your brain can't stand it so it escapes, it does anything to escape that feeling. Know what I mean?

KARRIE: Yes.

· THERAPIST: You need ways to handle that feeling so you have more options. That make sense? That's option 2—accept that you feel high emotion and help yourself without escaping into suicide thinking. That's crisis survival skills and radical acceptance, and a lot of turning your mind. The radical acceptance piece, I think (*Here therapist radically shifts her voice tone from matter-of-fact to deeply tender, slowing her pace of speech, with long silences between phrases.*), is your current relationship with your parents is a source of great pain . . . it is hard . . . it hurts deeply . . . Yeah?

KARRIE: (*Teary-eyed; nods.*)

THERAPIST: So, some of what we need here is acceptance, without flailing around and escaping the pain, yeah? So that's option 2, deeply accepting the intensity and high emotion, and helping yourself without escaping to suicidal thinking. (*Adds option 2 for therapy task on the whiteboard.*) OK, again, say it back to me, in your own words, OK? Like, "OK, I'm afraid of being humiliated. When that happens my brain always goes to suicide. That's my cue, I've got two options: (1) solve the problem so I don't get humiliated; (2) radically accept, help my physiology, regulate the emotion."

KARRIE: Yeah.

THERAPIST: OK, you put it in your own words. Right now you are doing the most important step. You're soothing your physiology, taking yourself seriously, working on the problem. Your turn. Put the whole thing together in your own words.

KARRIE: (*Restates in her own words, sipping her soda, counting her breaths.*)

THERAPIST: Which do you want to start with?

Task 5c: Intervene

Karrie chose to work first on planning to talk with her roommate and handle the job interview as best she could. This work went smoothly. When troubleshooting what to do in case things did not go well, the target naturally shifted to how Karrie can tolerate shame and humiliation if they fired. As was illustrated in Chapter 4, the therapist used validation to hold Karrie in brief, informal exposure episodes by discussing the meaning of having to ask her parents for help. The therapist used cognitive modification strategies to target Karrie's unrealistic expectations of herself and of asking for help. Because Karrie's skills group leaders were covering the emotion regulation skill of opposite action, she and Karrie easily incorporated the skill handouts for shame to determine whether shame was or wasn't justified and Karrie agreed to use this situation for her group homework assignment so that she could get help from the skills trainers, too. Further, the therapist used in-session contingencies: when

Karrie expressed her primary emotions the therapist was warm and supportive, but when Karrie escaped into statements about suicide or other extreme solutions, the therapist's voice tone became cool as she labeled each of such statements as escape. In sum, the therapist blended the four change procedures of skills training, exposure, contingency management, and cognitive modification to increase Karrie's ability to regulate shame without escape to intentional self-injury.

In the above session, the therapist followed the same basic sequence of assess, motivate, and move, over and over again. She also combined the core strategies of change, validation, and dialectics in various ways throughout the session. The exact mix of strategies varies to fit the moment, sometimes leaning to the dialectical, sometimes more to change or validation with the aim of making as much movement as possible in each interaction. The point is that many routes lead from point *A* to point *B*. Just as if you were taking a physical journey, on some routes the travel is easy, you can make great time. If you get a flat tire, or break down in some minimal way, there's a brief delay while you fix it. Highlighting and solution analysis are like this. Brief rifts in collaboration may be fixed easily with orienting, didactic strategies, or validation. Some terrain, however, requires a different vehicle like a mountain bike. At times, therapy tightly narrows to a nearly impassible footpath through the mountains, where you both are clawing your way on bloody knees. The going is slow and painstaking. Because you are balancing multiple priorities, you will need to remain flexible, and choose what works for where you are.

This can be difficult work. Integrating strategies to best balance acceptance and change requires skills we as therapists may lack. As well, the ability to regulate our own emotion in the face of complicated, high-risk problem behaviors that are slow to change may challenge us at the deepest professional and personal level. This is why the consultation team's role is crucial. The team helps the therapist develop and maintain the skills and motivation needed by applying all the treatment strategies discussed thus far to the therapist, as we'll see in the next chapter.

SEVEN

The Individual Therapist and the Consultation Team

Adequately caring for our clients can require more skill and emotional capacity than we have. When people are chronically suicidal and prone to emotion dysregulation, problems in the therapy and the glacial pace of change make treating the therapist as important as treating the client. In DBT, treating the therapist is required to adhere to the model. The team's purpose is to ensure each team member has the motivation and skill needed for this challenging work. This chapter illustrates how the DBT peer consultation team applies DBT to the therapist and how the therapist applies DBT to him- or herself.

We've all experienced case consultation where we describe the client and then we and our colleagues or consultant(s) look at the client material. It's as if we put an object on the table and all eyes focus on that object, the client. Sometimes when we present the client's case, our colleagues respond by discussing the problems intellectually, comparing theoretical approaches, or give us bland approval or overly critical feedback that leaves us dissatisfied and unhelped. Such environments often reward looking competent rather than disclosing where we struggle—we may leave looking good, but we're alone again and still stuck.

DBT peer consultation is different from that. Rather than a group of experts who come together to discuss the client as a case, the DBT consultation team is a group of peers who come together to work with each other with the same care, attention, and rigor of doing therapy with clients. *The therapist is the client.* The therapist puts *him- or herself* on the table, explicitly focusing on where she struggles to deliver high-quality DBT. The team works with the therapist to enhance his or her motivation and capability; the team applies DBT to the therapist. A well-functioning DBT team resembles an effective work group of scientific or artistic collaborators who come together to strengthen each other's work.

PURPOSE AND FORMAT
OF DBT CONSULTATION TEAMS

The typical DBT team has 6 to 8 members and meets for 60–90 minutes weekly or every 2 weeks. Members on a DBT team usually make two major commitments to each other. First, team members agree to participate in team meetings. Teams should clearly define the specifics of "participation" such as expectations about attendance, being on time, whether the therapist must carry individual DBT cases to be on the team, and so on. More importantly, teams should establish the general spirit behind agreeing to participate: to join the team means we agree to make every effort to increase our own and others' effectiveness as DBT therapists. In other words, the purpose of a DBT consultation team is to help team members apply the principles of DBT, not an alternative treatment. This means that while working together in consultation team members strive to help each other develop adherence and competence with DBT rather than offer ideas or debates from alternative models. In essence, the team agrees, during the meeting, to speak a common language and work from a shared model, even if therapists on the team may use other treatment models in other contexts.

"Making every effort" includes such basics as creating a nonjudgmental atmosphere for problem solving that encourages self-disclosure and self-critique, and each being open to give and receive sensitive, direct feedback. The norms of the group should mirror those of any therapy relationship where each member is taking care of the process of helping the client (in this case the therapist). Each member is actively listening. Each exerts the self-discipline to keep the conversational flow squarely focused on meeting the therapist's consultation needs, striving to be concise and reining in tangents. Participating means we agree to work to understand each other, especially in disagreements; we work in a matter-of-fact, proactive way to resolve problems that interfere with the team's process. For example, just as you would never consider it acceptable to be late for a therapy session or do your paperwork with a client or interrupt the session to text or take a call, so too the norm is that you participate with undivided attention and if something interferes, then you proactively figure out solutions to the problem. For example, if a team member arrived late

to a meeting, in a well-functioning team, that member would spontaneously self-assess the causes and generate solutions so it wouldn't happen
again, expecting to apologize and repair with his teammates with the
same respect he'd repair with a client. If this didn't spontaneously happen, a teammate might ask what happened and what the plan was, and
the therapist would nondefensively recognize and solve the problem.

Second, members agree to be responsible for the outcomes of *all* clients treated by the team, not just the ones they treat individually. The
implication here is that if a client seen by any therapist on the team com-
mits suicide, all therapists will say "yes" when asked if they have ever
had a client commit suicide. This commitment, much like the four-miss
rule for clients, activates team members to take responsibility to worry
and help solve problems. If members feel reluctant to make this commitment, it may indicate genuine problems that must be resolved for the team
to trust each others' work. For example, say a therapist solved the tremendous financial pressures arising from a complicated divorce by seeing more clients. She couldn't say no and took very high-risk clients. Her
beleaguered, defensive style blocked others from efforts to understand
exactly what she was doing and left her team worried. Without the commitment to share responsibility for all clients, most of us would opt for
a passive, respectful, "Well, I'll gently express my concerns, but I don't
want to intrude . . ." and then let the therapist struggle along, spread so
thin she could make serious mistakes that leave the team open to liability.
Sharing responsibility instead prompts a level of active problem solving
more like, "Carol, I'm worrying about you struggling to bear up under the
load you are carrying. I somehow want to help because anyone spread so
thin is bound to miss important things and we may end up with a suicide.
I don't want that to happen to you and I don't want that to happen to your
client and I don't want that to happen to me or the team, so somehow, as
respectfully as possible, the team needs to better see where you are struggling with these high-risk cases."

As in other modes of DBT, the team members make explicit agreements about how they will work together, beginning with these six consultation team agreements (Linehan, 1993a).

1. *Dialectical agreement.* We agree to accept a dialectical philosophy:
   There is no absolute truth. When caught between two conflicting
   opinions, we agree to look for the truth in both positions and to
   search for a synthesis by asking such questions as, "What's being
   left out?"
2. *Consultation-to-the-patient agreement.* We agree that the primary
   goal of this group is to improve our own skills as DBT therapists,

and not serve as a go-between for patients to each other. We agree to not treat patients or each other as fragile. We agree to treat other group members with the belief that others can speak on their own behalf.

3. *Consistency agreement.* Because change is a natural life occurrence, we agree to accept diversity and change as they naturally come about. This means that we do not have to agree with each others' positions about how to respond to specific patients nor do we have to tailor our own behavior to be consistent with everyone else's.

4. *Observing limits agreement.* We agree to observe our own limits. As therapists and group members, we agree to not judge or criticize other members for having different limits from our own (e.g., too broad, too narrow, "just right").

5. *Phenomenological empathy.* All things being equal, we agree to search for nonpejorative or phenomenologically empathic inter- pretations of our patients', our own, and each other's behavior. We agree to assume we and our patients are trying our best, and want to improve. We agree to strive to see the world through our patients' eyes and through one another's eyes. We agree to practice a nonjudgmental stance with our patients and with one another.

6. *Fallibility agreement.* We agree ahead of time that we are each fal- lible and make mistakes. We agree that we have probably done whatever problematic thing we're being accused of, or some part of it, and so we can let go of assuming a defensive stance to prove our virtue or competence. Because we are fallible, it is agreed that we will inevitably violate all of these agreements, and when this is done we will rely on each other to point out the polarity and move to a synthesis.

When a new member wants to join the team, take care to fully discuss how the team's purpose and format do and do not fit with the therapist's professional goals. The new member needs to agree and commit to ful- filling the obligations that come with joining the team. The team leader or person orienting the potential member (or sometimes even the entire team) should meet with the person to learn about his or her professional and personal goals as they relate to joining the team and explore how the team's purpose and ways of working do and do not align with those goals. Participation on a DBT team must be voluntary. Commitment strategies, troubleshooting, and other strategies may be used to strengthen commit- ment. Explicit commitments are made with the understanding that once made there is every expectation that the member will abide by those com- mitments.

Consultation Team Meeting Format

The consultation meeting itself begins with one member of the team assuming role of facilitator and leading a 5-minute mindfulness practice. The practice can be drawn from the DBT skills manual (Linehan, 1993b) or other sources. Because any activity can be done mindfully, you can also, if useful, tie practices thematically to the team's needs (e.g., for a team with members struggling with burnout anything from mindfully listening as a poem is read or mindfully free writing in answer to "Where are things hard for me clinically?" or "What do I need from today's consult?"). See Dimidjian and Linehan (2003) for excellent instructions on the essentials of teaching mindfulness in a clinical context. Here is an example (based on Salzberg, 2006) of a basic instruction:

> "Take a comfortable position, both feet on the floor, hands resting comfortably. As you sit comfortably you may hear external sounds, you may hear internal sounds, you may hear a certain quality of silence (*15–30 seconds of silence*).
>
> "As you hear sounds, notice the quality of your attention . . . the way the mind is present as you simply listen; the open, spacious quality. Noticing that the object of sound appears and we simply hear, simply listen. We don't have to make the sounds come or go. We don't have to define them or do anything about them in order to hear them, to connect. The object of sound appears and we're present, we connect to it. The mind can be relaxed, spacious (*pause 30 seconds*).
>
> "Now see if you can bring that same feeling tone, that quality of relaxed open spacious awareness to feeling the sensations of breathing, whereever you feel them most strongly. No need to make the breath deep or long or different from however it is and however it changes. Simply be aware of it, one breath at a time (*pause 10 seconds*).
>
> "If you find your attention wandering, in a very relaxed and patient manner, simply come back to sensations of breathing. I'll ring the bell three times now to start, and one time at the end to finish" (*all sit for 3–4 minutes*).

Team members then bring that mindful quality of attention forward into the meeting, much like a troupe of improv dancers or musicians, poised, alert, ready to do what is needed to work together to make a good experience. Each team member has gathered attention, and is ready to listen and create conditions that support the therapist's open disclosure of difficulty.

After mindfulness practice, the meeting facilitator asks members "Who needs consultation?," divvying up agenda time based on clinical needs and using the target hierarchy to prioritize the group's time just as one does in individual sessions. Teams have different ways of doing this, but the gist is that therapists who need help treating life-threatening behavior and imminent treatment dropout have first dibs on time, followed by those with other urgent consultation needs, team-interfering behavior and therapy-interfering behavior, and so on. Some teams leave this completely to the discretion of each therapist to ask for the amount of time that they need. Other clinics and training teams may need to know the status of all clients and so develop ways of quick report on high priority incidents (e.g., have a whiteboard on which are listed stage 1 targets and as each therapist enters the meeting, he lists his clients' initials to indicate who has had occurrence of that target since the last meeting).

Each therapist strives to arrive at the meeting prepared to succinctly describe the problem(s) he or she faces in delivering high-quality DBT. This lets the team get right to the heart of the consultation need, making the best use of their often limited time. In essence the therapist says, "I am here, I need to be there and I'd like your help in the following ways." For example, the therapist might say, "I need a clearer conceptualization," "I need help with ideas on the treatment plan" or "I am having trouble feeling empathy and I need help sorting out why" or "I want you guys to share this success my client had this week, so when I get hopeless next week, you'll remind me we have had a moment or two of progress!" Most often therapists need help assessing and thinking clearly about what is interfering with the therapy or what the client needs. All team members monitor the group's process to make sure the therapist's needs are met. The facilitator (or a designated timekeeper) keeps track of time.

HOW THE DBT CONSULTATION TEAM TREATS THE THERAPIST

The team treats each therapist who requests consultation as their client, applying DBT to help the therapist. As team members listen to their colleague, they use the same framework they use with clients: "Given where the person wants to go, what's getting in the way? What's going well?" "Is the person motivated? "What can we do to help move the therapist toward where she or he needs to be?" We use the same tools, too: chain analysis to determine controlling variables and combinations of highlighting, solution analysis and change procedure, validation, and dialectical strategies. Figure 7.1 outlines the steps that team members use in conceptualizing the consultation request and responding to it.

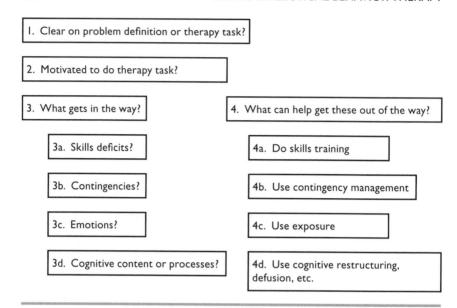

FIGURE 7.1. Conceptualizing where the therapist needs help.

The first move in consulting to a therapist is for the facilitator and team members to paraphrase the consultation question to check that they understand what the therapist needs. The consultation question needs to be clear. Sometimes all the therapist needs is a clearer problem definition and will know what to do once the issue is clarified. If not, then, just as with clients, team members apply behavior therapy assessment to see if the therapist has the motivation and skill needed to do the therapy task or solve the problem.

In some cases, the therapist just needs a little assistance with problem solving. The therapist describes the dilemma, and teammates offer solutions. For example, a therapist wanted to check if she had done enough troubleshooting, orienting, and commitment work needed with a new client. The client had a complicated relationship with her psychiatrist. She met weekly for 1-hour appointments, ostensibly for med management, and he'd stuck with her through many suicide crises as her other past therapists bailed out. The therapist expressed her concerns about the client having two simultaneous primary therapists and explored the client's willingness and reservations about the transition to the DBT program. The therapist summarized the highly collaborative conversation she and the client had had: the client understood the therapist's concern and together they thought through the transition. The client subsequently spoke with her psychiatrist, and reported back that the psychiatrist wholeheartedly agreed to the plan of relinquishing the individual therapist role and instead would solely provide medication management. A team member at this point observed, "This all sounds really good, but you still seem worried. What's worrying you?" The therapist said she didn't feel confident that the client accurately conveyed the plan nor could she trust the psychiatrist was really on board when all she had was the client's report. The team then suggested ideas of how the therapist might use consultation-to-the-client strategies to jointly write a letter to the psychiatrist and plan a follow-up phone meeting to ensure all roles were clear and all parties had agreed on how to handle crises. In this example, all that was needed was a little clarifying, validating the therapist's concern, and brainstorming on how to apply principles to generate solutions.

At other times, a skills deficit gets in the therapist's way. In that case, the team helps the therapist acquire, strengthen, or generalize the needed therapeutic skills. For example, the therapist may not know how to do a needed discrete therapy task such as assessing ADHD in an adult or creating an adequate safety plan for a client in a domestically violent relationship. The therapist may not know protocols for common co-occurring problems like panic attacks, social anxiety, or problem drinking. Or the therapist needs help generalizing interpersonal skills she does have in a new context (e.g., how to best break the news to a sensitive client that the therapist is pregnant and will take a maternity leave). Or the therapist may need some behavioral rehearsal. For example, the therapist might want modeling of how to coach a client who becomes dysregulated by shame and dissociates in session and then might role-play to practice and get feedback. Or a strongly change-oriented therapist may bring a tape cued to a difficult moment in therapy and ask for suggestions about how to validate rather than repeatedly moving to change the client.

Sometimes, the therapist has the skill but a combination of emotional reactions, contingencies, and cognitive content or processes interfere with the therapist using the skills. In this case, the team treats the therapist with the appropriate combination of change procedure(s). For example, a therapist asked for 20 minutes of consultation time because she was starting to dread phone coaching calls with one client. The team helped her identify the controlling variables setting off dread. The therapist quickly did a chain analysis of the problem using a coaching call from the previous night. She pinpointed the length of phone calls as a problem. Perceptive questions from her teammates helped her realize that she felt very guilty getting off the phone. This worked against keeping the call to her preferred 10-minute length. When the team and she assessed this moment in more detail, she saw that it was not only guilt that kept her on the phone. The client provided clear contingent consequences. When the therapist stayed on longer, it was positively reinforced by the client's genuine appreciation. Further, the client used the coaching and had averted many crises as a result. On the other hand, when the therapist ended the call in a timely way, the client communicated intense hurt and disappointment: staying on the phone was negatively reinforced by avoiding these aversive consequences. At this point, one teammate jumped in to say, "You need opposite action to unjustified guilt . . . just set the egg timer and hang up at 10 minutes on the dot!" The therapist flinched, feeling both irritated and shamed—the comment seemed to oversimplify the problem and imply that she should have already solved it. Another teammate read this reaction and stepped back to offer a problem definition: "So, the dilemma you have is that offering help as you have has really made many changes possible; the client wouldn't have been able to pull it off without that level of availability, and yet some of these times your own best interest, and therefore ultimately the client's best interests, would be for you to shorten the calls. Is that right?" The therapist said yes and then the facilitator added, "And another piece is that you already have a sense that at times guilt gets to you, so there are times when you'd rather have a nonguilty assessment of what is in the client's best interest in that moment."

With this problem definition and validation, the therapist felt understood and said, "Yes. It's that I don't feel free to get off the phone, I feel like I *have* to stay on, that's what's aversive. And then I judge myself for treating her as fragile, not being more firm and . . . (then, with a twinkle in her eye) I'm noting my own time now in consultation team's about up. How about this—I'll do some self-monitoring, gather some instances of when this happens, and start to do a solution analysis of where I can get this to go differently."

At the next meeting, the therapist used her time devising her treatment strategies to shape the client into more efficient phone calls. The strategies included more instruction in session to help the client organize her thoughts before she called, so that she could start by describing the problem and the list of skills she had already tried. The therapist had also used self-monitoring and started to notice a broader pattern of problematic coping with the discomfort of disappointing people. She had practiced pausing to be mindful of the sensations of guilt, rather than immediately jumping to resolve discomfort. The team role-played ending phone calls, over and over, in the face of disappointment to help desensitize the therapist. The team helped the therapist experiment with different exit lines, until she had an overlearned response. Both the individual therapist and the team take an active stance to solve problems that interfere with the therapist doing high-quality DBT.

Ensuring the Team Functions Well: Dealing with Common Problems

Time pressure requires the group to have tremendous skill as consultants. The conversation must stay focused despite the high complexity of the problems to be solved. Skill is needed when therapists feel high emotion, especially when corrective feedback is hard to hear and hard to give. Teams should pay attention to two sets of predictable trouble: the irritatingly human ways we get off track when discussing problems in groups and the inevitably conflict-avoidant and polarized responses we have when valid, divergent opinions arise.

Getting Off Track; Staying On Track

Focused group conversations are a rare thing—we've all been party to rambling unfocused meetings. Several irritatingly human habits interfere with useful consultation meetings. Ineffective consultation begins when the therapist poses an ill-formed consultation request, especially if the content or the therapist's manner sets off worry in teammates. Out of the desire to be helpful, team members often then jump in, usually with problem-solving suggestions before clarifying the request or assessing the problem. Even if the therapist is quite clear, it's natural for group discussion to wander here and there if team members aren't carefully tracking whether their comments are usefully focused on the problem at hand. Sometimes everyone's best efforts to stay clearly focused still aren't enough. This can happen when the problem itself is so complex that it is simply too difficult to talk through in a short time in a group. But the group may not realize this before four different legitimate directions have been proposed based on completely different conceptualizations of the problem. Time's up, and the therapist is left more confused than when he or she started.

This predilection to engage in behaviors that interfere with the consultation to the therapist has led Linehan to offer a set of things that help team members remember the key principles and spirit of consultation. For example, one team member can be assigned the role of "observer," and when he or she observes team-interfering behaviors he or she rings the mindfulness bell to cue the team to self-correct the process. Yet, most teams have difficulty self-correcting with insight alone. Before they can self-correct, they need to deliberately practice the components skills. For example, framing clear consultation questions leads to better-quality consultation because team members can see what help is needed. Therapists need to practice intentionally improving the clarity of their consultation requests and then seeking feedback by having the other team members paraphrase the request to see if the question was understood. Team members tend to simply jump to begin consulting without having checked they've correctly understood the consultation issue. Here again, team members deliberately can practice a sequence of routinely pausing to paraphrase the request to confirm what is needed, ask for clarification and, when the request is clear, *then* move into consultation. Similarly, teams sometimes jump into problem solving without assessment. Teams can practice by imposing the discipline of offering several comments that paraphrase, define the problem behaviorally, or otherwise validate the therapist or client before offering any ideas for solutions.

It's also not uncommon for team members to lose track of the original consultation request. The therapist asking for consultation and the facilitator take primary responsibility for remembering the precise consultation request and monitoring to make sure the conversation stays on track. The other team members should also monitor and check on whether the consultation is on track. While the conversational reins should stay in the therapist's hands, for the most part, it is unavoidably human to get pulled off track. The therapist may ramble into too much detail so the request gets lost; teammates may get caught up in their own line of thought. When the team or therapist drifts (as each inevitably will), whoever notices should gather the reins and put them back into the therapist's hands by rephrasing the original request or restating the working problem definition just as would be done in therapy with a client.

Here again, teams can benefit from deliberately practicing staying on track. After a person makes a consultation request, one or two people can be assigned the role of pulling the conversation off track. First, the therapist practices taking back the conversational reins by reasserting her needs, saying, "Guys, this is not on track for me—I need X." The therapist can practice "broken record" and other interpersonal effectiveness skills to pull the team back into a helpful consultation. A variation is to have the *therapist* be the one who derails the conversation by becoming tangential, too detailed, frustrated, or emotionally withdrawing after someone's comment. Then the facilitator or other teammate can practice correcting the process. This is done by restating the original consultation question or paraphrasing the current working problem definition and then handing the conversation back to the therapist by asking if this focus is on track. Especially on larger teams or teams that carry high case loads, there is seldom time to waste belaboring a point, even when it's valid. Teams often need practice exerting self-discipline and returning again and again to the larger purpose of meeting the therapist's consultation needs.

Working with Divergent Views:
Returning to a Dialectical Stance

When the therapist has said, "I am here but I need to be there," another teammate may have a divergent view on what is happening in the therapy and what needs to be done about it. Because each therapist controls the agenda during his or her consultation time, he or she can say, "Thanks, I hadn't thought of it that way" and work with the team member's idea. Alternatively, he or she can say, "Thanks. That's off track for this reason . . . " The latter response demonstrates that the therapist has taken the point into consideration, but finds it more helpful to direct the conversation to something else. The beauty of a team is that many divergent views are offered; in fact, the client has six or eight talented therapists for the price of one. However, there are times when a member, many members or the leader, see something that they believe is important to address but the therapist disagrees. Useful divergence threatens to become rigid polarization.

In the case of Yvette, described in Chapter 5, her therapist met with the consultation team between getting Yvette's mumbled phone message about her self-harm and Yvette's next session. As the therapist began to ask for consultation, a less experienced team member who worked in Yvette's day treatment program offered nonempathic explanations for her behavior. He told a story of watching Yvette hear "No" from one nurse and then charm another into saying "Yes" to get a painkiller for a migraine. His tone implied that the therapist was a bit naïve not to see what a "manipulative person" Yvette was. The use of dialectical stance and strategies in the team interaction came into play. The therapist "stepped in where angels fear to tread" and simply described her experience in a nonjudgmental, matter-of-fact tone, "I don't feel helped by that story. I don't see her as manipulative and me as naïve not to see it. I don't want to spend the brief time I have for consultation on that." A more experienced person on the team stepped forward, "Ah, yes, it's about time we got polarized around here! Looks like you've both got a different bit of the elephant. But, given you (nodding to the therapist) are in a crisis with the elephant, tell us again what you want help with?" Another member offered a definition of the consultation problem: "If I were you I'd need time to get my thinking organized, because you are trying to coach her through a suicide crisis without her going into the hospital, right? How would it be if you lead us through your thinking and then tell us where you need help?"

When team members get polarized, as in the above example, the team members need to remember they are treating the therapist. They should do what is needed to rein in judgmental or off-track comments, help the therapist re-regulate if needed, and redirect all team members back to an effective problem-solving conversation. In general, it helps for the team to institute practical steps to keep the conversation usefully divergent rather than unhelpfully polarized. One way to do this is to read the consultation agreements at the beginning of each meeting, or at least one agreement, as a reminder of the guidelines the team has agreed to follow (Linehan, 1993a). Another useful idea is to quite actively validate divergent views by paraphrasing until you get a head nod from the person that you have understood their point of view. When a case is highly complicated it can be helpful to further structure the conversation by having team members ask to take control of the floor, having one person speak at a time, using the whiteboard to visually represent the divergent viewpoints, and constantly insisting the group return to understanding and validating divergent views.

How the Team Treats Therapists' Therapy-Interfering Behaviors

The most important way team members help each other is to point out behavior that interferes with therapy that they cannot see for themselves. Therapists' personal problems or foibles may become significant barriers to their work with their clients or in team. Therapist issues with depression and chronic pain, distraction with overloaded lives, habitual ways of coping or regulating emotion can compromise the care that the therapist can give and may reasonably become a target for the team.

The problem, of course, is that we all have difficulty speaking up when we think our colleagues are problematic. We don't say anything. For example, a therapist comes in describing the irritating sporadic attendance of her client and how the client comes so late (when she bothers to show at all) that the only thing they have time to target is her attendance problem. The therapist reminds the team that the same problem has gotten the client fired many times from work and from prior therapies. She concludes by saying it may be time to let her drop out of the program. The team, having been along for the ride, remembers that the client's problems with attendance began after the therapist had sporadic attendance herself due to health problems and doctor appointments. The teammate who knows the therapist best has noted that the therapist's irritability, physical pain, and low-grade depression have affected their friendship. The therapist has been less warm and less emotionally present and the colleague suspects this has also affected the therapeutic relationship. The natural human tendency is to avoid talking about "the elephant in the room"— the probability that the therapist has played some part in the client's poor attendance and consequently might need to change herself to get change in the client.

Many things make it hard in these situations to speak as freely as needed. First, we often do not feel we have consent to offer direct negative feedback. Second, therapists are a sensitive lot! If you want to distress a therapist, tell him he is not helping his patients. If we have a concept of ourselves as "good therapists," feedback otherwise can be threatening. This then leads to the next problem, created by the lack of time. If you offer critique of a colleague's work, whether phrased skillfully or inadvertently not so skillfully, it may land badly. Your colleague resists your feedback, tells you you're off base or indirectly communicates she's hurt or angry. Of course you want to clarify, someone else jumps in, and around you go, often not quite straightening it out. Eventually, one of you capitulates saying, "Oh, it's fine. Let's go on." But these things are often not fine and produce resentment. It is hard to bring it up again without seeming defensive, yet you can't let it go. If it's not safe to give honest feedback then there will be no true intimacy, risk taking, or growth, or the team will eventually come to a rift. Members exit.

All of this can be even harder when the person who needs the hard-to-hear feedback is the team leader. When a team leader is the most senior, knowledgeable person, teammates don't give needed feedback even though the leader is open to feedback. Team members may doubt they have anything useful to add; they may defer to the leader's greater expertise or they may genuinely not have new ideas beyond what the leader has already thought of. At other times, the leader may not take feedback well and have difficulty removing the "leader hat" to truly be a clinical peer during a consultation meeting. Countering these natural obstacles takes concerted effort, from the team leader and members; they must learn to tolerate discomfort in the service of providing needed feedback. Team leaders in particular may find it helpful to have an outside consultant with whom to discuss cases and who may even attend team meetings and comment on how to improve consultation.

Despite the natural human tendency to avoid in these difficult situations, it is not an option on a DBT team. We share responsibility and clinical risk. The skills we need to practice as consultants are the same needed with sensitive clients and we find ways to work on treatment-interfering behavior collaboratively and dialectically. Validation and stylistic strategies make all the difference in these circumstances when giving and receiving tough feedback. All members need the skill of being able to highlight something problematic in a light, easy manner, and to describe nonjudgmentally. The person asking for consultation needs to be assertive, and in particular assert a nondefensive "broken record" that asks for honest critique and demonstrates resilience so colleagues will not pull their punches. For example, "Tell me what you think I am doing that is problematic? . . . OK, what else could I improve? . . . Great, anything else you see that needs work?"

Let's return to the therapist with health problems who has a client with problematic attendance. After listening, a teammate says in a genuine, kind voice, "Wow, she is so incredibly frustrating! It's hard to even remember she is doing the best she can." This provokes the most irreverent person on the team to say, with perfect deadpan, "Why do we let these people with problems in here, anyway?" The whole team, along with the therapist, bursts into laughter. As the belly laughs subside, another teammate steps in where angels fear to tread and using a completely nonjudgmental tone, says, "Mary, I notice I'm hesitating to ask you if your health absences are impacting the client's attendance, but I don't want to treat you as fragile, you know, assume you'd be defensive. So, I wonder, maybe you can say how that might be playing a part, too." Here the therapist is being invited to look nonjudgmentally and nondefensively at herself and is expected to step up to the challenge. Other team members also have a part to play—to not step in to rescue the therapist. If the therapist's body posture next communicates that she can't handle it, others need to demonstrate nonjudgment and solidarity by using validation and self-disclosure. At this point, someone might say, "You know, it makes me think about how I lost Marla to dropout when my teenager was having all that trouble with school . . . I think as a team we don't have a good way of working with these folks with sporadic attendance, especially when the therapist needs help hanging in there."

However, despite the team's efforts as the discussion continued, the therapist did respond defensively, saying how much harder her life had become and how impossible it would be for her to extend her limits and do all the outreach needed to pull the client back in. The team then became polarized, with some feeling the team was being too hard on the therapist to even have this conversation, while others were concerned for the client, insisting that some real treatment plan be implemented rather than letting her drift out of the program. At a particularly tense moment, one team member said, "Listen, I don't want to be harsh, but I feel like we need to be real here, and it has been incredibly hard to see you suffer through these health concerns. You have been a pillar of this team. And I had not got it until today how hard this has been and I feel terrible about that. You need help here and I can pick up a group or even pick up a transfer case next month." The therapist responded, "I'm just feeling too defensive to hear you. I am not an invalid!" The team held its collective breath, everyone tense. The elephant in the room had been named. Then the trusty irreverent person said, "No, you're not an invalid, you're a Ferrari that suddenly finds yourself trapped in a Toyota body, trying somehow to keep up with your Mazerati of a client on the speedway . . . I don't know, I'm scared for you and for her, my friend. I feel like we need to get the pace car out there and slow things down and really think about what your actual not-as-healthy limits are and what that means for your treatment plan with her." With great tenderness, he said, "We gotta figure this out. We can't let you keep pretending you have your old stamina and nothing is wrong. We're a team and we need to pitch in somehow. And we can't let her drop out without a fight. What do you want the next step to be?"

The therapist said she wanted to think about it; it was hard to stay open, but she trusted the team. That week the therapist met with her own therapist, who verified the team's take: she was neither fully present nor working within her body's capacity. In her own personal therapy, she began the painful work of accepting the effect of her declining health and thought through the new limits she needed in order to work at her best. She decided to reduce her practice by half and work only in the morning. Then in her next meeting with her client, the therapist shared the way she believed her health had been impacting their therapy negatively. As she spoke honestly about her own limits with the client, they began to problem solve and negotiate to determine what changes each could make to solve the problems with poor attendance. Even as the client understood and appreciated the therapist's need for morning appointments, it became clear that this was a hardship for the client since she worked the night shift. It would take months to make a schedule change at her workplace. At various points in the conversation, the client became extremely dysregulated by fear and by anger at the therapist, responding with hopeless and passive statements. When this happened, the therapist soothed, validated, and treated the dysregulation while continuing to problem-solve around the unwelcome limits her health now imposed on them both. Despite their efforts they reached an impasse—the therapist's limits did not work from the client's perspective. While there are times where it is indicated for the therapist to extend limits, at least temporarily, this was not a viable solution in this case. The therapist expressed her genuine wish that her health and limits were different as she continued to feel deeply committed to the client, but the client withdrew into a cool matter-of-fact resignation. The therapist described what she viewed as maladaptive escape, validated that the client might be too hurt and angry and fearful at the moment, and wondered if perhaps meeting with her favorite skills trainer for a session or two to think through her options would be better than the client's current urge to completely toss in the towel on the whole program. This eventually resulted in the client successfully transferring to a new therapist although not without significant wear and tear on all parties.

What is important to note here is that in DBT the process of observing limits is a real relationship negotiation rather than a set of arbitrary rules. The therapist notices the impact of the client's behavior and her own life circumstances, and then, the two must—just as in any relationship—work through both parties' needs and desires as best they can. In the above case example, client and therapist were not able to reach a mutually acceptable arrangement yet the separate outcomes for each were much more positive than if the problems had been ignored. These outcomes were made possible by the team's ability to consult well with dialectically balanced, profound validation and urgent challenges to change.

HOW THERAPISTS APPLY DBT TO THEMSELVES

Therapists repeatedly experience difficult emotions in the course of clinical work with clients and outside of session. Difficult emotions may be prompted by the client's behaviors and circumstances (e.g., the sheer tragedy in our clients' lives), or by our own therapeutic errors, failures to observe limits, and personal history. The habitual ways we regulate and fail to regulate emotion can accumulate into a sense of burnout. As is true for clients, many of our therapy-interfering behaviors then stem from our difficulty regulating emotion. For example, at the end of a session, a client told the therapist that he doubted the therapy was having any effect. The therapist was not clear whether to view this as important feedback, an instance of the client's problem (i.e., hypothesized it functioned as escape), or both. The therapist asked a number of questions to understand the controlling variables for the client's comment. This resulted in the therapist losing track of the time and ending the session late. Ending late in turn meant the therapist had to race to make her son's baseball game. She arrived late, missing the home run he hit in the first inning. Sitting in the stands, with the emotional fallout from the afternoon's events, the therapist struggled to enjoy the game.

In DBT, you actively treat your therapy-interfering behaviors by using the DBT skills and by applying the treatment principles to yourself. You begin with self-monitoring. It need not be formal or fancy—sometimes the back of the envelope or tally marks on a Post-it note are sufficient. In the vignette above, for example, the therapist had noticed feeling demoralized with a few clients and began tracking instances of difficult emotion related to her work and how she coped with them. Figure 7.2 shows one example of the self-monitoring sheet she used. After she reviewed several weeks of self-monitoring, she identified two related problems. First, the common denominator across situations was that she wasn't sure how to understand and respond to client's hopeless statements, particularly in the face of slow or minimal treatment progress. This had the biggest negative emotional impact on her when it happened at the end of the day when she was tired. Second, she saw that her efforts to cope with her

Date: May 10	Situation: Last session of day; Z (client) dropped hopeless statement about lack of progress; went late trying to understand concerns (missed J's home run)
Difficult private reactions (e.g., thoughts, feelings, sensations)	Irritated; "Do I need this?"; confused, insecure; "He needs a better therapist"; tense in pit of my stomach
Distress/disturbance level (when it first happened)	Not distressing/ disturbing Extremely distressing/ disturbing 1 2 3 ④ 5
Coping strategy (my response to my private reactions)	Fantasize about quitting work; mad at myself for letting myself be late to game—thoughts about how typical this is; shame/discouragement—I should be better at this; try to leave it behind and enjoy evening
Short-term effects	Not at all effective Incredibly effective 1 2 ③ 4 5
Long-term effects	Not at all effective Incredibly effective ① 2 3 4 5

FIGURE 7.2. Coping strategies diary entries. Based on Hayes (2006).

difficult emotions were only marginally effective and left her in the same basic spot: a repetitive struggle of subtly blaming herself or her client in the face of slow change. She needed a mini-treatment plan to minimize the emotional wear and tear that sapped her energy for clinical work. She sketched out two chain analyses looking first for controlling variables for her client's hopeless statements and second, for controlling variables for her own problematic responses to these statements. To generate solutions for these problems, she took what she knew of these chain analyses to her treatment team. The team's brainstorming generated a list of highly practical solutions for the therapist's therapy-interfering behavior as shown in Figure 7.3.

As can be seen in this example, DBT therapists actively practice skills from all DBT skills modules. In many clinical situations, change is impossible or difficult and slow and the therapist needs skills to accept and embrace the moment as it is. Therefore, in DBT, you (the therapist)

Chain Analysis Vulnerability Factors	Solution Analysis Alternative Responses w/Client
End of day, tired	• Observe and describe "right in the moment" • Adopt default phrase "What you are saying feels important to me, too important to rush through at the end when we have no time." Then plan when and how to discuss.
Prompting Event(s)	
Client makes hopeless statement, indicates therapy isn't helping	
	• Use as cue to review the treatment plan, including consultation from team to address my own doubts regarding treatment effectiveness.
Links	
Confusion/Doubt	
1. Is this a problem or progress for this particular person?	• Clarify case conceptualization—how does this behavior function for this client?
2. Is therapy having an effect?	• On son's game days: reschedule to see only easy clients; use the last hour to do paperwork rather than see client.
Targeted Problem Behavior	
Jump into assessing or problem solving, lose track of time; worry and ruminate unproductively; escape distress without doing anything that reduces the likelihood of this loop happening again	Alternative Responses w/Myself • Observe and describe the actual experience of confusion and doubt as my daily mindfulness practice each time it occurs.
Consequences	• Radically accept that doubt and confusion are part of the work.
Highly intermittent reinforcement by client expressing more hope—just like a Las Vegas slot machine!	• On hard clinical days, increase self-care.

FIGURE 7.3. Chain and solution analysis of therapist's therapy-interfering behavior.

practice the core mindfulness skills, willingness, turning the mind, radical acceptance, and exercises to cultivate awareness. DBT does not require that the therapist have a formal meditation practice (e.g., seated meditation for 45 minutes each day in addition to the brief formal mindfulness that begins each DBT consultation team meeting). At a minimum, however, DBT therapists should practice skills enough for their teaching to be based on experience using skills, not just intellectual understanding (Dimidjian & Linehan, 2003, p. 427). While longer sessions of formal practice are optional, my own opinion is that the therapist's practice of mindfulness skills grounds everything we do as a DBT therapist: in each interaction, you practice observing, describing, and participating (act intuitively from wise mind) while practicing being nonjudgmental (neither good nor bad), one-mindful ("in the moment"), and effective (focused on what works).

Use of mindfulness, radical acceptance, and awareness skills can take many forms in the context of clinical work. Fulton (2005) makes the point that the influence or incorporation of mindfulness by the therapist ranges from the implicit influence of the therapist's own mindfulness practice to the explicit use of mindfulness with clients. On the implicit side, he says, mindfulness practice may cultivate greater ability to attend and concentrate, to feel compassion and empathy, and to see suffering from a larger perspective. The DBT therapist connects, again and again, with her client and her own experience, with open, spacious attention, noting and letting go of habitual judging, grasping, and avoiding. The therapist deliberately practices in order to cultivate the qualities of mind to meet all experience with a welcoming, friendly stance, like the sun shining on all things equally. The therapist practices all the time with awareness of the breath while listening, half-smiling while listening, observing and describing nonjudgmentally what you notice happening as you interact (Linehan, 1993b). (Many great resources are coming out for therapists; see also Wilson & DuFrene, 2008.)

Sometimes mindfulness practices are used in combination with other skills. For example, in session one therapist found himself irritated by the client's behavior of arriving 20 minutes late without calling to notify him of the delay. Knowing he could have had 20 minutes to return calls and catch up on charting that were instead wasted checking the waiting area rankled him. As the client began to explain, the therapist used opposite action to downregulate the intensity of his irritation by validating aloud to the client all the ways the client's behavior could not be otherwise. Being mindful of his emotion, and knowing that anger is typically a secondary reaction for him, the therapist noticed the primary emotions were disappointment and worry. Softening, he then described his disappointment to the client and together they talked through how to get the situation to go differently next time.

At other times, the therapist might deliberately bring mindfulness to understanding subtle factors that may be contributing to therapy-interfering behavior. For example, a therapist had two clients communicate that they felt looked down on and humiliated when with him, although neither could identify what set off that feeling. This was incredibly distressing for the therapist whose intent and actual feeling was quite the opposite. He role-played a typical sequence with a teammate, both of them pausing frequently to reflect on their experience. The colleague's ability to notice and describe nonjudgmentally identified that when the therapist felt interest, he straightened his posture and narrowed his focus to a laser beam—on the receiving end it felt like scrutiny, a light so bright that there was no place to hide. The therapist's usual warmth also became much more difficult to experience. Mindful attention in their interaction during the role-play allowed the therapist to identify a subtle but nevertheless quite powerful personal habit that negatively impacted his clients. With this insight, and influenced by the thinking and preliminary research from Gilbert (2009), he then readily made changes to increase his verbal expression of warmth, slow his pace, and actively adopt a gentler, soothing body posture to balance the narrowing of attention that happened so strongly in him when the emotion of interest or strong curiosity fired up.

Sometimes, the therapist treats her therapy-interfering behavior with radical acceptance. For example, as shown on Figure 7.3, the therapist who was struggling with burnout began to use her difficult reactions as the object for mindfulness practice. She noticed over time the predominance of self-doubt and how often her mind jumped around like an agitated monkey whenever self-doubt appeared. Without pathologizing it, she simply watched what Fulton (2005) called the "self-congratulatory pendulum"—when her clients were doing well, she felt great; when they were doing poorly, it "ruined her mood." It was quite predictable, boringly predictable in fact, after watching it for several weeks. Then a teammate led a mindfulness practice of listening to the rain, one wet dreary Seattle Friday, with storms predicted all weekend. He set up the practice by telling the story of how his brother was in town, for the first time in years, and they had planned to play golf on the public course as they had as kids. But here he was, in a different moment than he hoped for. All morning he'd been listening to the rain and practicing radical acceptance and he invited the team to join him. He would listen to the rain and when he noticed himself fighting the moment, he would make a silent mental note, "Yes, this is how it is right now: raining." He described simply feeling the sensations of the lump in his throat and constricted breathing as disappointment welled and he made the silent mental note, "tightness," "sadness." He described noting the thoughts and objections and planning that arose with a simple "also here now." He drew the parallel to their clinical work, "If you work with people who really suffer, it hurts. You will feel confused, powerless, defeated—many, many difficult emotions—it rains here where people suffer." The team practiced together for several minutes listening to the rain and radically accepting whatever came with the silent mental note "and this, too."

The therapist adapted this radical acceptance practice to use at the end of each workday. She would look at her calendar for 5 minutes, briefly calling to mind each client to "see if it rained"—that is, to feel and accept how it was for her, radically accepting whatever was difficult just for what it was. Then to end the practice, she'd send a smart, kind smile to her heart. "This is how it is right now."

Grounded in this practice of radical acceptance, the therapist's change-oriented coping strategies took on a feeling tone of ease. Even her escapist fantasies about leaving the field changed. The therapist began to use those thoughts as an indicator light: when they turned on, it meant something problematic was happening. What set them off? The therapist also used them as hints about what pleasurable activities she might explore to better balance her life. The frequency of difficult emotions did not change much but the stance of "It's all good; whatever the moment offers can be worked with," was incredibly freeing to her. In the most fundamental sense, members of a DBT consultation team strive to develop their skills and emotional capacity.

This spirit of consultation, that of a community of therapists treating a community of patients, all in it together, characterizes the best DBT teams. All in the same human boat, doing the best we can with what we have been given. More alike than different, as we feel vulnerable, as we suffer, and as we find our way. In the most radical sense, when we are with our clients and teammates in the hardest moments, we feel "There, but for the grace of God, go I."

References

Allen, L. B., McHugh, R. K., & Barlow, D. H. (2008). Emotional disorders: A unified protocol. In D. H. Barlow (Ed.), *Clinical handbook of psychological disorders* (4th ed., pp. 216–249). New York: Guilford Press.

Antony, M. M., & Barlow, D. H. (Eds.). (2010). *Handbook of assessment and treatment planning for psychological disorders* (2nd ed.). New York: Guilford Press.

Barlow, D. H., Farchione, T. J., Fairholme, C. P., Ellard, K. K., Boisseau, C. L. Allen, L. B., et al. (2011). *The unified protocol for transdiagnostic treatment of emotional disorders: Therapist guide.* New York: Oxford University Press.

Beck, A. T., Rush, A. J., Shaw, B. F., & Emery, G. (1979). *Cognitive therapy of depression.* New York: Guilford Press.

Becker, C. C., & Zayfert, C. (2001). Integrating DBT-based techniques and concepts to facilitate exposure therapy for PTSD. *Cognitive and Behavioral Practice, 8,* 107–122.

Bohart, A. C., & Greenberg, L. S. (Eds.). (1997). *Empathy reconsidered: New directions in psychotherapy.* Washington, DC: American Psychological Association.

Cloitre, M., Koenen, K. C., Cohen, L. R., & Han, H. (2002). Skills training in affective and interpersonal regulation followed by exposure: A phase-based treatment for PTSD related to childhood abuse. *Journal of Consulting and Clinical Psychology, 70,* 1067–1074.

Crowell, S. E., Beauchaine, T. P., & Linehan, M. (2009). A biosocial developmental model of BPD: Elaborating and extending Linehan's theory. *Psychological Bulletin, 135,* 495–510.

Dimeff, L. A., & Koerner, K. (Eds.). (2007). *Dialectical behavior therapy in clinical practice: Applications across disorders and settings.* New York: Guilford Press.

Dimidjian, S., & Linehan, M. M. (2003). Mindfulness practice. In W. O'Donohue, J. E. Fisher, & S. C. Hayes (Eds.), *Cognitive behavior therapy* (pp. 229–237). New York: Wiley.

Ebner-Priemer, U. W., Badeck, S., Beckmann, C., Wagner, A., Feige, B., Weiss, I., et al. (2005). Affective dysregulation and dissociative experience in female patients with borderline personality disorder: A startle response study. *Journal of Psychiatric Research, 39*, 85–92.

Fairburn, C. G. (2008). *Cognitive behavior therapy and eating disorders.* New York: Guilford Press.

Feeny, N. C., Zoellner, L. A., & Foa, E. B. (2002). Treatment outcome for chronic PTSD among female assault victims with borderline personality characteristics: A preliminary examination. *Journal of Personality Disorders, 16*, 30–40.

Foa, E. B., & Kozak, M. J. (1986). Emotional processing of fear: Exposure to corrective information. *Psychological Bulletin, 99*, 20–35.

Foa, E. B., Hembree, E. A., Cahill, S. P., Rauch, S. A. M., Riggs, D. S., Feeny, N. C., et al. (2005). Randomized trial of prolonged exposure for posttraumatic stress disorder with and without cognitive restructuring: Outcome at academic and community clinics. *Journal of Consulting and Clinical Psychology, 73*, 953–964.

Foa, E. B., Riggs, D. S., Massie, E. D., & Yarczower, M. (1995). The impact of fear activation and anger on the efficacy of exposure treatment for posttraumatic stress disorder. *Behavior Therapy, 26*, 487–499.

Foa, E. B., Rothbaum, B. O., Riggs, D., & Murdock, T. (1991). Treatment of posttraumatic stress disorder in rape victims: A comparison between cognitive-behavioral procedures and counseling. *Journal of Consulting and Clinical Psychology, 59*, 715–723.

Frijda, N. H. (1986). *The emotions.* London: Cambridge University Press.

Fruzzetti, A. E., Santisteban, D. A., & Hoffman, P. D. (2007). Dialectical behavior therapy with families. In L. A. Dimeff & K. Koerner (Eds.), *Dialectical behavior therapy in clinical practice: Applications across disorders and settings* (pp. 222–244). New York: Guilford Press.

Fulton, P. R. (2005) Mindfulness as clinical training. In C. K. Germer, R. D. Siegel, & P. R. Fulton (Eds.), *Mindfulness and psychotherapy.* New York: Guilford Press.

Gladwell, M. (2008). *Outliers: The story of success.* New York: Little, Brown.

Goldfried, M. R., & Davison, G. C. (1976). *Clinical behavior therapy.* New York: Holt.

Goldfried, M. R., Burckell, L. A., & Eubanks-Carter, C. (2003). Therapist self-disclosure in cognitive-behavior therapy. *Journal of Clinical Psychology, 59*, 555–568.

Golier, J. A., Yehuda, R., Bierer, L. M., Mitropoulou, V., New, A. S., Schmeidler, J., et al. (2003). The relationship of borderline personality disorder to posttraumatic stress disorder and traumatic events. *American Journal of Psychiatry, 160*, 2018–2024.

Greenberg, L. S. (2002). *Emotion-focused therapy: Coaching clients to work through their feelings.* Washington, DC: American Psychological Association.

Harned, M. S., & Linehan, M. M. (2008). Integrating dialectical behavior therapy and prolonged exposure to treat co-occurring borderline personality disorder and PTSD: Two case studies. *Cognitive and Behavioral Practice, 15*, 263–276.

Hart, J. (2007). *A writer's coach: The complete guide to writing strategies that work*. New York: Anchor Books.

Hayes, S. C. (2006). *Get out of your mind and into your life*. Oakland, CA: New Harbinger.

Hayes, S. N., & O'Brien, W. O. (2000). *Principles of behavioral assessment: A functional approach to psychological assessment*. New York: Plenum/Kluwer Press.

Hembree, E. A., Cahill, S. P., & Foa, E. B. (2004). Impact of personality disorders on treatment outcome for female assault survivors with chronic posttraumatic stress disorder. *Journal of Personality Disorders, 18*, 117–127.

Izard, C. E. (1991). *The psychology of emotions*. London: Plenum Press.

Jaycox, L. H., & Foa, E. B. (1996). Obstacles in implementing exposure therapy for PTSD: Case discussions and practical solutions. *Clinical Psychology and Psychotherapy, 3*, 176–184.

Juengling, F. D., Schmahl, C., Hesslinger, B., Ebert, D., Bremner, J. D., Gostomzyk, J., et al. (2003). Positron emission tomography in female patients with borderline personality disorder. *Journal of Psychiatric Research, 37*, 109–115.

Koons, C. R., Robins, C. J., Tweed, J. L., Lynch, T. R., Gonzalez, A. M., Morse, J. Q., et al. (2001). Efficacy of dialectical behavior therapy in women veterans with borderline personality disorder. *Behavior Therapy, 32*, 371–390.

Linehan, M. M. (1993a). *Cognitive-behavioral treatment of borderline personality disorder*. New York: Guilford Press.

Linehan, M. M. (1993b). *Skills training manual for treating borderline personality disorder*. New York: Guilford Press.

Linehan, M. M. (1996). Dialectical behavior therapy for borderline personality disorder. In B. Schmitz (Ed.), *Treatment of personality disorders* (pp. 179–199). Germany: Psychologie Verlags Union.

Linehan, M. M. (1997a). Behavioral treatments of suicidal behaviors: Definitional obfuscation and treatment outcomes. In D. M. Stoff & J. J. Mann (Eds.), *Neurobiology of suicide: From the bench to the clinic* (pp. 302–328). New York: Annals of the New York Academy of Sciences.

Linehan, M. M. (1997b). Validation and psychotherapy. In A. Bohart & L. Greenberg (Eds.), *Empathy reconsidered: New directions in psychotherapy* (pp. 353–392). Washington, DC: American Psychological Association.

Linehan, M. M., Armstrong, H. E., Suarez, A., Allmon, D., & Heard, H. (1991). Cognitive-behavioral treatment of chronically parasuicidal borderline clients. *Archives of General Psychiatry, 48*, 1060–1064.

Linehan, M. M., Bohus, M., & Lynch, T. R. (2007). Dialectical behavior therapy for pervasive emotion dysregulation. In J. Gross (Ed.), *Handbook of emotion regulation* (pp. 581–605). New York: Guilford Press.

Linehan, M. M., Comtois, K. A., Murray, A. M., Brown, M. Z., Gallop, R. J., Heard, H. L., et al. (2006). Two-year randomized controlled trial and follow-up of dialectical behavior therapy vs. therapy by experts for suicidal behavior and borderline personality disorder. *Archives of General Psychiatry, 63*, 757–766.

Linehan, M. M., Dimeff, L. A., Reynolds, S. K., Comtois, K., Shaw-Welch, S., Heagerty, P., et al. (2002). Dialectical behavior therapy versus comprehensive validation plus 12-step for the treatment of opioid dependent women meeting criteria for borderline personality disorder. *Drug and Alcohol Dependence, 67,* 13–26.

Linehan, M. M., Heard, H. L., & Armstrong, H. E. (1993). Naturalistic follow-up of a behavioral treatment for chronically parasuicidal borderline clients. *Archives of General Psychiatry, 50,* 971–974.

Linehan, M. M., Schmidt, H., III, Dimeff, L. A., Craft, J. C., Kanter, J., & Comtois, K. A. (1999). Dialectical behavior therapy for clients with borderline personality disorder and drug-dependence. *American Journal of Addiction, 8,* 279–292.

Linehan, M. M., Tutek, D. A., Heard, H. L., & Armstrong, H. E. (1994). Interpersonal outcome of cognitive behavioral treatment for chronically suicidal borderline clients. *American Journal of Psychiatry, 151,* 1771–1776.

Lynch, T. R., Cheavens, J. S., Cukrowicz, K. C., Thorp, S. R., Bronner, L., & Beyer, J. (2007). Treatment of older adults with co-morbid personality disorder and depression: A dialectical behavior therapy approach. *International Journal of Geriatric Psychiatry, 22,* 131–143.

Lynch, T. R., Morse, J. Q., Mendelson, T., & Robins, C. J. (2003). Dialectical Behavior Therapy for depressed older adults: A randomized pilot study. *American Journal of Geriatric Psychiatry, 11*(1), 33–45.

Lynch, T. R., Trost, W. T., Salsman, N., & Linehan, M. M. (2006). Dialectical behavior therapy for borderline personality disorder. *Annual Review of Clinical Psychology, 3,* 181–205.

Marlatt, G. A., & Donovan, D. M. (Eds.). (2005). *Relapse prevention: Maintenance strategies in the treatment of addictive behaviors* (2nd ed). New York: Guilford Press.

McDonagh, A., Friedman, M., McHugo, G., Ford, J., Sengupta, A., Mueser, K., et al. (2005). Randomized trial of cognitive-behavioral therapy for chronic posttraumatic stress disorder in adult female survivors of childhood sexual abuse. *Journal of Consulting and Clinical Psychology, 73,* 515–524.

Meadows, E. A., & Foa, E. B. (1998). Intrusion, arousal, and avoidance: Sexual trauma survivors. In V. M. Follette & J. I. Ruzek (Eds.), *Cognitive-behavioral therapies for trauma* (pp. 100–123). New York: Guilford Press.

Miller, A. L., Rathus, J. H., DuBose, A. P., Dexter-Mazza, E. T., & Goldberg, A. R. (2007). Dialectical behavior therapy for adolescents. In L. A. Dimeff & K. Koerner (Eds.), *Dialectical behavior therapy in clinical practice.* New York: Guilford Press.

Nock, M. K. (2009). Why do people hurt themselves?: New insights into the nature and functions of self-injury. *Current Directions in Psychological Science, 18,* 78–83.

O'Donohue, W., & Fisher, J. E. (Eds.). (2009). *Cognitive behavior therapy: Applying empirically supported techniques in your practice* (2nd ed.). Hoboken, NJ: Wiley.

Porr, V. (2010). *Overcoming borderline personality disorder: A family guide for healing and change.* New York: Oxford University Press.

Rittel, H. W. J., & Webber, M. M. (1973). Dilemmas in a general theory of planning. *Policy Sciences, 4,* 155–169.

Robitschek, C. G., & McCarthy, P. R. (1991). Prevalence of counselor self-reference in the therapeutic dyad. *Journal of Counseling and Development, 69*(3), 218–221.

Rogers, C. R., & Truax, C. B. (1967). The therapeutic conditions antecedent to change: A theoretical review. In C. R. Rogers, E. T. Gendlin, D. J. Kiesler, & C. B. Truax (Eds.), *The therapeutic relationship and its impact: A study of psychotherapy with schizophrenics* (p. 101). Madison: University of Wisconsin Press.

Rosenthal, M. Z., Cheavens, J. S., Lejuez, C. W., & Lynch, T. R. (2005). Thought suppression mediates the relationship between negative affect and borderline personality disorder symptoms. *Behaviour Research and Therapy, 43,* 1173–1185.

Safer, D. L., Telch, C. F., & Agras, W. S. (2001). Dialectical behavior therapy for bulimia nervosa. *American Journal of Psychiatry, 158*(4), 632–634.

Salzberg, S. (2006). *Insight meditation: A step-by-step course on how to meditate.* Sounds True Press.

Shenk, C., & Fruzzetti, A. E. (2011). The impact of validating and invalidating responses on emotional reactivity. *Journal of Social and Clinical Psychology, 30,* 163–183.

Stiglmayr, C. E., Grathwol, T., Linehan, M. M., Ihorst, G., Fahrenberg, J., & Bohus, M. J. (2005). Aversive tension in patients with borderline personality disorder: A computer-based controlled field study. *Acta Psychiatrica Scandinavica, 111,* 372–379.

Telch, C. F., Agras, W. S., & Linehan, M. M. (2001). Dialectical behavior therapy for binge eating disorder. *Journal of Consulting and Clinical Psychology, 69*(6), 1061–1065.

Tomkins, S. (1963). *Affect, imagery and consciousness: The negative affects.* New York: Springer.

Tomkins, S. (1983). Affect theory. In P. Ekman (Ed.), *Emotion in the human face* (pp. 137–154). New York: Cambridge University Press.

Truax, C., & Carkhuff, R. (1967). *Toward effective counseling and psychotherapy.* Chicago: Aldine.

Tsai, M., Kohlenberg, R. J., Kanter, J., Kohlenberg, B., Follette, W., & Callaghan, G. (2009). *A guide to functional analytic psychotherapy: Awareness, courage, love and behaviorism.* New York: Springer.

van den Bosch, L. M., Koeter, M. W., Stijnen, T., Verheul, R., & van den Brink, W. (2005). Sustained efficacy of dialectical behaviour therapy for borderline personality disorder. *Behaviour Research and Therapy, 43,* 1231–1241.

Verheul, R., van den Bosch, L. M., Koeter, M. W., de Ridder, M. A. J., Stijnen, T., & van den Brink, W. (2003). Dialectical behaviour therapy for women with borderline personality disorder: 12-month, randomised clinical trial in the Netherlands. *British Journal of Psychiatry, 182,* 135–140.

Wagner, A. W., & Linehan, M. M. (1997). Biosocial perspective on the relationship of childhood sexual abuse, suicidal behavior, and borderline personality disorder. In M. Zanarini (Ed.), *The role of sexual abuse in the etiology of borderline personality disorder* (pp. 203–223). Washington, DC: American Psychiatric Association.

Wagner, A. W., & Linehan, M. M. (2006). Applications of Dialectical Behavior Therapy to PTSD and related problems. In V. Follette & J. Ruzek (Eds.), *Cognitive-behavioral therapies for trauma* (2nd ed., pp. 117–145). New York: Guilford Press.

Wilson, K. G., & DuFrene, T. (2008). *Mindfulness for two: An acceptance and commitment approach to mindfulness in psychotherapy.* Oakland, CA: New Harbinger.

Wright, J. H., Basco, M. R., & Thase, M. E. (2006). *Learning cognitive-behavior therapy: An illustrated guide.* Washington, DC: American Psychiatric Publishing.

Zanarini, M. C., Frankenburg, F. R., Dubo, E. D., Sickel, A. E., Trikha, A., Levin, A., et al. (1998). Axis I comorbidity of borderline personality disorder. *American Journal of Psychiatry, 155,* 1733–1739.

Zanarini, M. C., Frankenburg, F. R., Hennen, J., & Silk, K. R. (2004). Mental health service utilization by borderline personality disorder clients and Axis II comparison subjects followed prospectively for 6 years. *Journal of Clinical Psychiatry, 65,* 28–36.

Zanarini, M. C., Frankenburg, F. R., Reich, B., Hennen, J., & Silk, K. R. (2005). Adult experiences of abuse reported by borderline clients and Axis II comparison subjects over six years of prospective follow-up. *Journal of Nervous and Mental Disease, 193,* 19–27.

Zayfert, C., DeViva, J. C., Becker, C. B., Pike, J. L., Gillock, K. L., & Hayes, S. A. (2005). Exposure utilization and completion of cognitive behavioral therapy for PTSD in a "real world" clinical practice. *Journal of Traumatic Stress, 18,* 637–645.

Zimmerman, M., & Mattia, J. I. (1999). Is posttraumatic stress disorder underdiagnosed in routine clinical settings? *Journal of Nervous and Mental Disease, 187,* 420–428.

Zinbarg, R. E., Craske, M. G., & Barlow, D. H. (2006). *Mastery of your anxiety and worry: Therapist guide* (2nd ed.). New York: Oxford University Press.

Index

Page numbers followed by *f* and *t* indicate figures and tables, respectively.